BEEF IT!
Upping the Muscle Mass

BEEF IT!

Upping the Muscle Mass

by Robert Kennedy

editor of MuscleMag International

Sterling Publishing Co., Inc.   New York
Distributed in the U.K. by Blandford Press

Dedicated to Hardcore Iron Pumpers the World Over

Library of Congress Cataloging in Publication Data

Kennedy, Robert, 1938-
  Beef It! : upping the muscle mass.

  Includes index.
  1. Bodybuilding.   I. Title.
GV546.K46   1983   646.7'5   83-17887
ISBN 0-8069-4170-7
ISBN 0-8069-7760-4 (pbk.)

Third Printing, 1983

Copyright © 1983 by Robert Kennedy
Published by Sterling Publishing Co., Inc.
Two Park Avenue, New York, N.Y. 10016
Distributed in Australia by Oak Tree Press Co., Ltd.
P.O. Box K514 Haymarket, Sydney 2000, N.S.W.
Distributed in the United Kingdom by Blandford Press
Link House, West Street, Poole, Dorset BH15 1LL, England
Distributed in Canada by Oak Tree Press Ltd.
% Canadian Manda Group, P.O. Box 920, Station U
Toronto, Ontario, Canada M8Z 5P9
Manufactured in the United States of America
All rights reserved

CONTENTS

FOREWORD

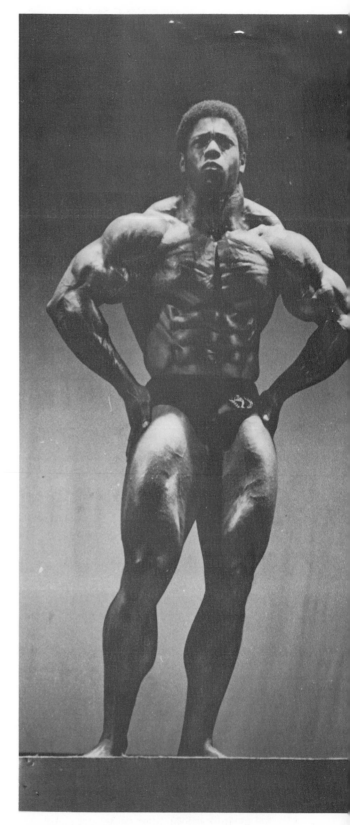

Bertil Fox—his fans yelled "Beef It!"—and he did!

Here we go again! My last book, *Hardcore Bodybuilding*, took off with a huge gust. Sales went sky high, and for the first time in my life I found myself on a best-seller list. I flew with the eagles—a glorious experience—but brought my head down from the clouds again in order to write this new tome. *Beef It!* digs deeper into the sport of bodybuilding than I have ever dared to before.

You may be thinking, why ever did he call his new book *Beef It!?* Well, I'll tell you. I heard this phrase for the first time during a bodybuilding contest in London, England. It was the 1978 NABBA Mr. Universe, in which two superb bodybuilders, Serge Nubret of France and Bertil Fox of England, were competing against each other. Fox was a former pupil of the older Nubret and had learned a few tricks on contest preparation. The comparison was difficult. Nubret had the more aesthetic physique—wide shoulders and narrow hips. His posing was tidy and elegant. In contrast to him Fox was massive. He lacked the Greek-sculpture beauty of Nubret but was endowed with pure rippling muscle from head to toe. The judges were in a quandary as to which type of physique to honor. Should they pay homage to beef or beauty?

As the two super-athletes posed down, Bertil's army of home-town London fans started to cheer for him. Somehow the chant became, "Beef it, Bertil!" On and on it went, "Beef it, Bertil! Beef it!" and pretty soon the judges were unanimous: they would pay homage to beef that day.

Backstage, after the judging, the despondent Nubret turned to a well known English photographer and with his thick French accent asked: "What ees thees 'Beet eet'? I don't understand." The photographer had to explain that the audience was chanting "Beef it," not "Beet eet." Then he enlightened Nubret about the meaning of this phrase. "Beef it," he said, "means 'pose to show maximum muscle, and forget about grace and beauty.' "

Now let me tell you about some of the chapters in this book.

I got a tremendous kick out of writing the chapter on power thinking (psychoblast). The mental side of bodybuilding is still in its infancy, but the champions acknowledge that we can become what we can picture clearly in our minds. Conversely, if we cannot visualize ourselves bathed in bodybuilding glory, then we will just not attain that state, now or at anytime in the future.

Chapter 13, the section on nutrition is, I believe, as scientific and helpful to the aspiring bodybuilder as anything previously seen in print. Not to be missed!

For reasons of space, I could do little more than touch on the subject of posing in *Hardcore Bodybuilding*. In this book you are holding, there is a lot of practical information on physique display—page after page of it.

Recuperation is another important aspect of training that requires analyzing and probing. I have tried to do just that in order to come up with the right answers. The rewards you will get from following my sage advice may amaze you and will certainly delight you.

In addition to getting into the specifics of training individual body parts, I devoted one chapter to structuring your routine for maximum results, and another chapter to body typing and what that means in terms of progress and success.

I can predict with 95 percent certainty that the chapter on the sticking point (Chapter 14) will be of immediate interest to you. Am I a clairvoyant? Sorry to say I am not, but it's a fact that at any one time 95 percent of all bodybuilders are in a rut.

Another important section of this book deals with training the metabolism (Chapter 12), for there are a great many trainers whose metabolism is out of kilter and should be adjusted.

Then there is bodyfat percentage. What? You don't want to hear about that now? In that case I'll just mention that you can find a chapter on it in this book, and you may be surprised at how low you can get yours!

Of course, there are many more chapters than that. The point I really want to make is that *Beef It!* starts where *Hardcore Bodybuilding* left off. If you liked *Hardcore*, then you'll like *Beef It!* If *Hardcore* taught you something, there's more for you here in *Beef It!*

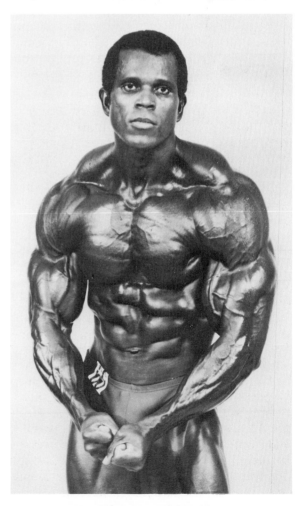

Serge Nubret—France's top physique.

7

Appreciation

Having just blown my own horn about the contents of this book, it is now time to humble up my act and give credit where credit is due. In the first place, there are the bodybuilders who appear in these pages. I have the greatest respect for them. They know what real training and preparation involves. They live the reality. I only write about it. My thanks and appreciation to each and every one of them.

To IFBB chief Ben Weider, who has actively helped me in my endeavors, I offer my hand in gratitude. His job of controlling and guiding world bodybuilding is seldom fully understood or acknowledged, but as my involvement with it has grown, so has my knowledge of Ben's service to this cause.

The photographers have each brought something unique to this book. There's Denie, a widely diversified photographer who is always ready, willing, and able to get the exact picture I want. Garry Bartlett, too. He's a laugh a minute, but serious when it comes to photography. Nothing of any importance goes unrecorded when Garry has his camera with him.

As always, Chris Lund's magic lens has played an important part in the appeal of this book. His photographic classics all bear his hallmark of being sharper than sharp. Other photographers to whom I owe many thanks include the indomitable Bill Reynolds; the world's most beautiful grandmother: Doris Barrilleaux;

Monty Heron; Art Zeller; Joe Valdez; John Balik; Roger Shelley; Bob Gruskin and Al Antuck, both of New York; Jim Marchand; and British camera artist, the late George Greenwood.

I am more than grateful to the gym owners who allowed my photographers to do their thing. Even when their gym floor was crowded and they had plenty of other problems, they smiled graciously and allowed the cameras to add to the confusion. To Pete Grymkowski and his partners at Gold's, to Ken Wheeler of Canada's Super Fitness Chain, to Joe Gold of World's Gym in California, and to a host of others who have shown both concern and kindness, a heartfelt thank you!

Finally, I would like to extend my appreciation to my editor, Jo Kaufmann, for her considerable input into bringing my manuscript into its final publishable state, and to Jim Anderson, whose design brought it all together.

If you are new to bodybuilding or haven't done any formal exercise for some time, get your doctor's OK before you begin. Ask for a stress test. After you've been checked over, you will be quite confident in maximizing your progress with an all-out effort. If by chance you do have some physical irregularity, then this examination will enable you to get some suitable treatment to correct the problem. Bodybuilding is for those who are in vigorous good health. If you are, smile. This book is for you!

1
MOTIVATION AND GOAL SETTING
Defining Your Wants

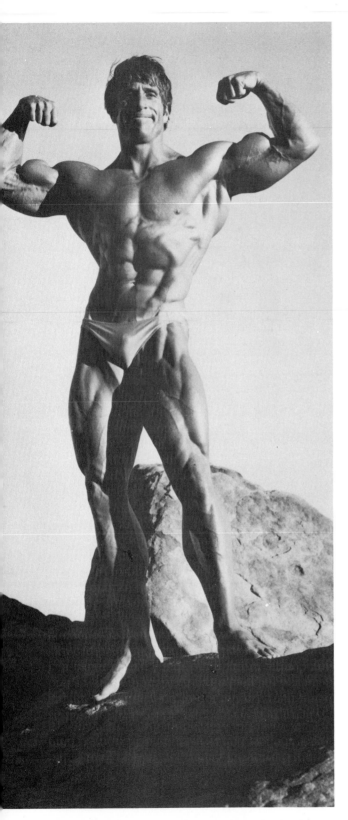

Steve Davis uses every motivational trick in the book to build his magnificent body.

Motivation is what drives you forward, more than any other thing. If you have it, whoopee! You are a driven man. You are hooked on bodybuilding, and nothing can hold you back. The gas pedal is locked in the down position, and all you have to do is steer.

I well remember my younger days when I, too, was a *driven* man. Bodybuilding was the only thing in my life. Nothing else mattered. I would not lift anything if it wasn't either a dumbbell or a barbell. Reading? No way—unless it was about muscles. Conversation? Only on the subject of bodybuilding. Yes, sir, in those glorious misspent days, I would turn down dates, wedding invitations, trips, hikes, anything, all because of the possibility of missing a precious, almost sacred workout. How I cursed the bodybuilding magazines of the day for insisting that one should only train three times a week. Why, I could have trained six hours daily every day!

If you are now as driven as I used to be, half your training battle is won. There is danger, of course. You could become a victim of uncontrollable enthusiasm. You could overwork, overtrain, become totally disillusioned, and ultimately give up in disgust. But it's far better to be overinspired and overmotivated than not to be inspired at all. Let that fire and longing burn deep within your bones. You need success. Nothing, nothing, nothing else matters!

With this inborn desire it is never a matter of whether you should train or not. The question doesn't arise. You wouldn't miss a workout if you were paid. The only question is how to make your workouts as useful, efficient, and beneficial as possible.

This inborn drive is often referred to as aggression. Author Denie, the former editor of *Muscle Training Illustrated*, goes one step further. He believes that the successful bodybuilders, the top champions, are often one step beyond that of being driven. "They are," says Denie, "enthusiastic and obsessive to the extent of being emotionally disturbed individuals."

Publisher Joe Weider states: "I have always believed that people who take up bodybuilding are the doers of the world. Given an outlet for their energy and creativity, they will build monuments."

Whatever the case, thank God for your motivation. Use your drive carefully, however. You have a very positive sense of self-assertiveness, but you must temper it with intelligent application to correct training. Otherwise? Whooosh! Burn-out City!

Utilize your aggression, because chances are that as you mature (heaven forbid!), your aggression will gradually desert you. And when motivation goes, you are in the unenviable position of having to drum up your enthusiasm artificially. You might also lose your attention-span for training. Sure, you still want the great-looking body, but the verb *want* is very different from the verb *need!*

Sometimes, this aggressive desire leaves a bodybuilder when he finds a steady girl friend. Sometimes it happens when financial independence arrives. Can you imagine saying, "Oh, no! I have been left a million dollars. Now I will never make it as a top bodybuilder!" Remember how tennis genius Bjorn Borg's "killer instinct" vanished when he got married? It doesn't always work this way, of course. Jimmy Connors got more fired up *after* marriage!

It is almost inevitable, however, that your *need* for huge muscles will gradually diminish with the advancing years. You will never lose it

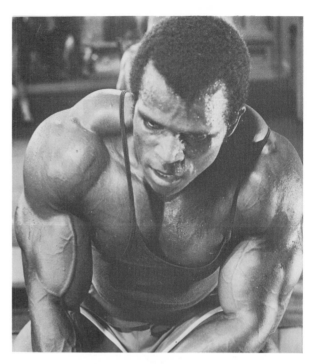

Setting specific goals is important to Serge Nubret.

completely, but believe me, it lessens—enough to result in less assertive workouts, missed training sessions, and less gym discipline.

Regardless of whether you have an uncontrollable need or only a wholesome want, you must organize your mind through a series of goal-setting actions. Without any positive and clearly visualized goals, you simply cannot succeed.

If you are not self-motivated, you must motivate yourself. Many people, bodybuilders included, remain satisfied with too little. Do not be content with insignificant achievements. Many get so far and no further. Do not be content with developing a body so that it's just a little better than the average physique. Lack of drive is death. Apathy is your enemy!

As a bodybuilder, you must not rest on your laurels. You must make every effort to cultivate the positive emotional force which compels the necessary physical action to take place, and the first essential is a positive, forceful mental outlook. You need to develop the attitude to life that does not accept permanent limitation. You must possess a spirit of abounding enthusiasm and the determination that ultimately makes failure impossible.

Forget the scoffers who say you are wasting your time. They are only showing their own lack of spirit and may well be envying yours.

Forget those who say, "Even if you succeed, it's not worth it!" You have enough on your plate without letting these negative thinkers weaken your resolve the least little bit.

It can be helpful at times to feel a certain amount of dissatisfaction; not the dissatisfaction of despair, but a dissatisfaction with your present level of achievement. You can use this as fuel for forging ahead, trying harder, and achieving success. Never fall into the trap of being satisfied with too little.

Bernarr MacFadden, known as the Father of Physical Culture, was frequently heard to say, "Without a goal, you will *never* succeed." He should know. He was a physical marvel until well into his eighties, and by that time he had built up a publishing empire worth millions of dollars.

I like John Balik's down-to-earth approach to goals and attitudes: "Goal-setting is the answer to the question: where am I going? Without clearly defined goals, short and long term, your journey through bodybuilding's waters will be like a ship without a destination. You must take the time and thought to clearly define your direction." John Balik is a writer and photographer for Joe Weider's *Muscle and Fitness Magazine* and knows all aspects of training and nutrition. His superstar nutrition manuals are particularly informative.

With regard to goal-setting, Balik says: "You have to understand your potential, and remember that every action starts as a thought. Without that first step, nothing is possible." According to Balik the three key questions you should ask yourself are:

1. What do I want out of bodybuilding? More weight? Leaner physique? Better proportions? Ultrafitness? To win Mr. Olympia?

Andreas Cahling uses the mind to further his progress.

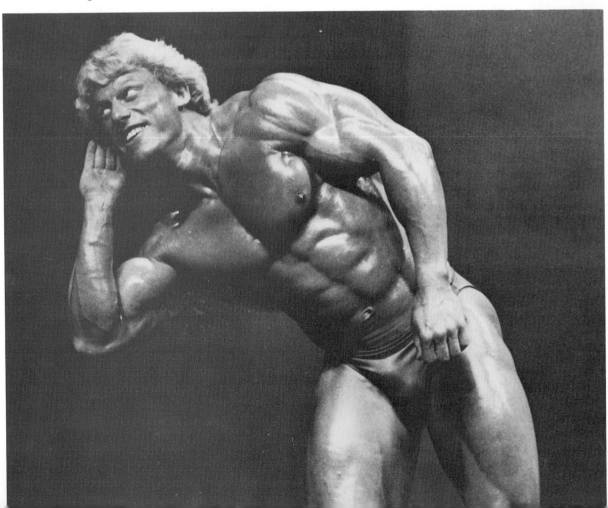

2. What body type am I? An endomorph (heavy-set and fat), a mesomorph (big boned and muscular), or an ectomorph (small-boned and skinny)?

3. What is the level of my experience?

As a beginner, you should aim to bench-press your bodyweight six times, and squat with your bodyweight for fifteen reps.

As an intermediate, you should aim for one and a half times your bodyweight for both six reps and for fifteen reps in the full squat.

When you get into advanced bodybuilding, you have to set your goals one month at a time. Write them down, and post them on your notice board where you can see them every day. That will continually remind you of where you want to be. Reinforcing your goals on a regular basis will help to steer your actions.

If your present training has not worked sufficiently, then instant change is necessary. Re-motivate yourself. Set realistic goals, and power your way with manly determination all the way to the top!

Arnold Schwarzenegger was one of the first of the modern set of bodybuilders to talk about visualization and goal-setting. Talking to Ken Dychtwald of *New Age Magazine*, Arnold lets us into his unique way of thinking on the subject:

Arnold's size is evident even when he is completely relaxed. This photo was taken by Robert Nailon just before they had a workout together.

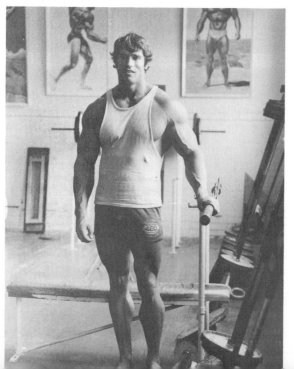

"When I was very young, I visualized myself as being there (at the top of bodybuilding) having achieved the goal already. Mentally, I never had any doubts in my mind that I would make it. I always saw myself as a kind of finished product out there, and it was just a matter of following through physically.

"But mentally I was there already. It makes it so easy, because then when you train for hours a day, you don't question yourself anymore. 'What am I doing here?' You focus right in again on your vision, on your image of what you know you will be, and that's why you're in the gym each day, to get a step closer to your goal.

"When I trained my biceps, I pictured huge mountains, much bigger than biceps can ever be. Just these enormous things. You do something to your mind in order to do certain things. I know my biceps aren't mountains—although they may look like miniature mountains. But *thinking* that they are gets my body to respond.

"When weightlifters are standing in front of a barbell, they must, in their minds, lift it in order to then lift the weight physically. If they have even one percent of doubt in their minds, they won't do it. When they stand before the bar and they close their eyes, what they are doing is lifting the weight mentally. And if they fail to lift it mentally, then they won't make the lift at all. Sure they may try. They go through the motions so that they can't be accused of not having a go . . . but it comes down to the same thing. Grunts and groans and ultimately a missed lift.

"Before a workout I would flex my muscles to get in touch. I locked my mind into my muscle during training, as if I'd transplanted my mind into the tissue itself."

An offshoot of visualization, and closely related to it, is the art of positive thinking. There are always people who will try to drop you down. When people are on a diet, some kind friends will be trying to get them to eat. It can be the same with training. People are sure to come up with all sorts of reasons why you shouldn't go to the gym today. Forget them. Surround yourself with positive, vibrant people. Right now you are bound for success. See the trail ahead, and allow nothing to get in your way. Do not let some negative thinker derail your journey to bodybuilding stardom. Keep your head straight. Deviate for no one. Have the courage to be the one in a thousand who breaks the bodybuilding barrier.

2
SOMATOTYPING
Do
You
Need It?

Serge Nubret, primarily a mesomorph, though he has very small wrists.

All men are created equal—or so the saying goes. Certainly, many people assume that, if for no other reason than they have heard it so often. It is supposed to be true in terms of the law, but cannot be claimed with respect to people's physical attributes.

Think of your various friends. Can you honestly say that all or any of them were created equal? One has a keener mind; another has more natural strength; and yet another may possess better mental and physical attributes than the other two. Each of us has a unique set of genes which endows us with some advantages *and* some disadvantages.

Way back some four hundred years before the birth of Christ, Hippocrates broadly classified human beings into four different types: the choleric, the sanguine, the phlegmatic, and the melancholic. This classification was expanded in 1797, by the Frenchman Halle; but today most people use the physique classifications, or somatotypes, established by Dr. William H. Sheldon of Harvard University, a leading exponent of anthropometry.

After extended work with thousands of subjects, Sheldon concluded that there were only *three* distinct body types, though he acknowledged readily that most people were really a mixture of these types. The following are the three physical types identified by Sheldon:

Endomorphs

Endomorphs have a rounded, pear-shaped physique, and a tendency to be fat. They have a wide thorax and a long, rounded abdomen. Their small intestine is 23–25 feet long, and their large intestine 5–8 feet. Thus their food has a much greater distance to travel than it would with other body types, and therefore endomorphs derive more nourishment from their food than the other types do. Most endomorphs have a placid, cheerful disposition, large bones, and a weight problem that probably started in childhood.

Mesomorphs

As far as bodybuilding goes, mesomorphs are the lucky ones. They are adept at strength sports, naturally muscular, and have a forceful appearance. They are staid, reliable, and normal in their habits and dietary requirements. In bodybuilding circles they are known as "quick gainers."

Ectomorphs

Ectomorphs have egg-shaped heads and angular features, and most of them are bundles of energy. Long and gangly, they usually don't have the slightest trace of fat. (Their small intestine has a length of only 10–15 feet.) Thin bones are their trademark, the rib cage is long, and at the thorax the angle is narrow. Having efficient lungs, they make natural long-distance runners.

Champions

By now you are wondering whether you have to be a mesomorph to get to be Mr. Olympia. Actually, no Mr. Olympia, past or present, has been a pure mesomorph, but they all have a large mesomorphic component in their makeup.

Bertil Fox and Frank Zane have different body types, yet each has built a great body.

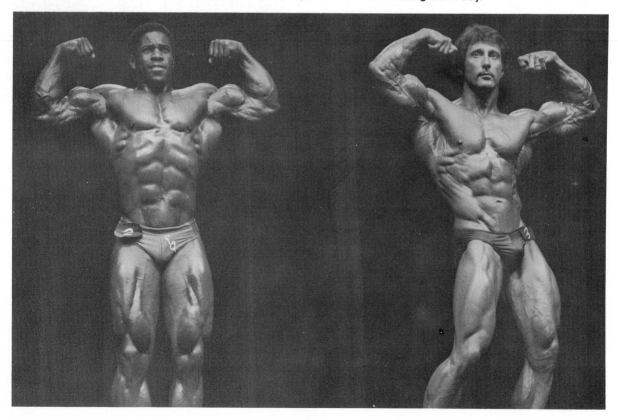

In real life, pure body types are rare. Most are a mixture of the three body types, though one of the types may be dominant. So Sheldon devised a numbering system for showing the degree to which an individual represents each of the three types.

The degree is expressed in numerals ranging from 1 to 7, with 1 denoting the lowest degree, and 7 the highest. A person's somatotype is then expressed in three numbers. The first number denotes the degree of *endomorphy* (roundness and fat). The second number denotes the person's *mesomorphy* (muscle, bone, and strength). The third number indicates the degree of *ectomorphy* (fragile bones, high energy, and low body-fat).

To illustrate that, let us consider a few famous physiques:

John Grimek

John shows a moderate degree of the first (endomorphic) component, probably 3. He is undoubtedly very high in mesomorphy, having large, square bones (wrist well over 8 inches), excellent muscular attachments, and a high muscle-cell count. Even without training, he would have fairly large muscles. His mesomorphic rating is about 6 or 7. He is very low in ectomorphy. There is very little of the long-distance runner type about him. He would rate no higher than 1 in ectomorphy. Grimek is probably a 3–6–1. He has a markedly dominant mesomorphic component.

Frank Zane

Zane is not a dumpy, round pear-shape, so his endomorphic component is obviously minimal. He gets a 1 in the endomorphic first category. His muscularity has always been evident, even from the earliest days of his training. I rate him 6 in the mesomorphic category. As for his ectomorphic component, Zane shows some evidence of a fine bone structure, though it is not fragile. Let's rate him a 2. Altogether then, Zane approximates the somatotype 1-6-2. Again, the mesomorphy ranks very high.

Mike Mentzer

I rate Mike a 2 for his endomorphic component. Not that he has anything like a pear shape, but his bones are very thick-set, and there is some slight inclination towards "thick skin." His

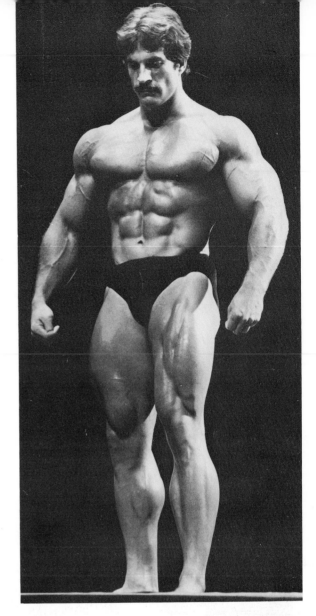

Mike Mentzer, one of the most genetically gifted bodybuilders.

abdomen is long from the thorax. His mesomorphic rating, to my mind, is monumental. He must be a 7. Mike has muscles from head to toe. I think you will also agree that Mentzer shows very little evidence of the thin, nervous ectomorphic component. I rate Mike Mentzer 2–7–1 somatotype.

Tony Pearson

Looking at Tony Pearson can be a little deceiving. He has mountains of muscles, but also has characteristic features of an ectomorph. He shows no evidence of the endomorphy at the opposite end of the scale. He does, however,

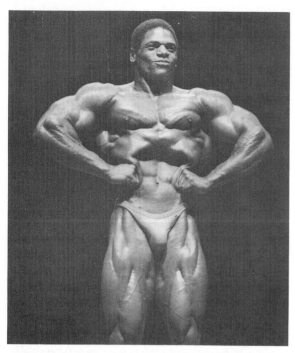

Tony Pearson could be described as light-boned, but look at the incredible body he has built!

have the broad-shouldered, naturally muscular appearance of the mesomorph, though not to the same degree as Mike Mentzer. I rate the incredible Tony Pearson as a 1–6–3.

Arnold Schwarzenegger

Rating Arnold is no easy task. He has the round head and general thickness of an endomorph, the muscle insertions and masculine excellences of a mesomorph, and some of the sensitivity of an ectomorph. I may be wrong, but I see Arnold as a 2–6–2.

The Uses of Somatotyping

You have seen now that it is not difficult to somatotype an individual. On the other hand, one cannot get an accurate picture of someone by just knowing the three numerals which denote his physical makeup. In other words, somatotyping gives us no more than a rough idea of a person's physical structure.

No doubt, the question of whether a person can change his somatotype by training or diet has come to your mind. I suspect that the official medical pronouncement would be that your basic type cannot be changed.

However, in the many years I have been associated with bodybuilders and bodybuilding, I had occasion to observe many structural changes that came about through regular training. There is no doubt that bones grow to accommodate muscle gains. I have also seen the basic shape of the thorax change after a few steady months of weight training.

Have you ever seen someone who has lost a great amount of fat? Somehow, even though you may never have seen them when they were overweight, you nevertheless *know* that they were heavy once. The reason for this is that, even though you see them now in their slimmed-down state, their bones have not yet shrunk. Somehow, their bones look too big for the amount of weight the individual is now carrying. Bone growth during the gain size period—whether it be fat, muscle, or both—is relatively slow. When you lose weight, the skeletal muscles are equally sluggish in returning to their previous, smaller dimensions.

Many years ago, the bodybuilding fraternity was persuaded by an unending series of articles and advertisements in popular bodybuilding magazines of the day that an aspiring bodybuilder could not possibly make gains in muscular size and strength unless he knew his exact body type, and tailored his training exactly to his particular classification. The advertisements would require the pupil to submit (along with a sizeable check) front, back, and side photographs, together with a photo depicting his abdominal retraction (his thorax with the waist sucked in to show the shape of the lower ribs). The more "straight across" the ribs appeared, the more endomorphic the pupil was; the narrower the angle, the more ectomorphic. Guided by that, the mail-order trainer would custom design a schedule to get the maximum results for the specific body type.

It's my opinion that too much emphasis was placed on the importance of this body-type classification. Physique classification has several practical uses. It indicates an individual's hereditary makeup and therefore his potential for physical improvement. It also indicates the sport at which he is most likely to excel, but it is not a key to exactly how a person should train (how many sets, reps, or exercises). Nevertheless there are certain guidelines the specific types should adhere to.

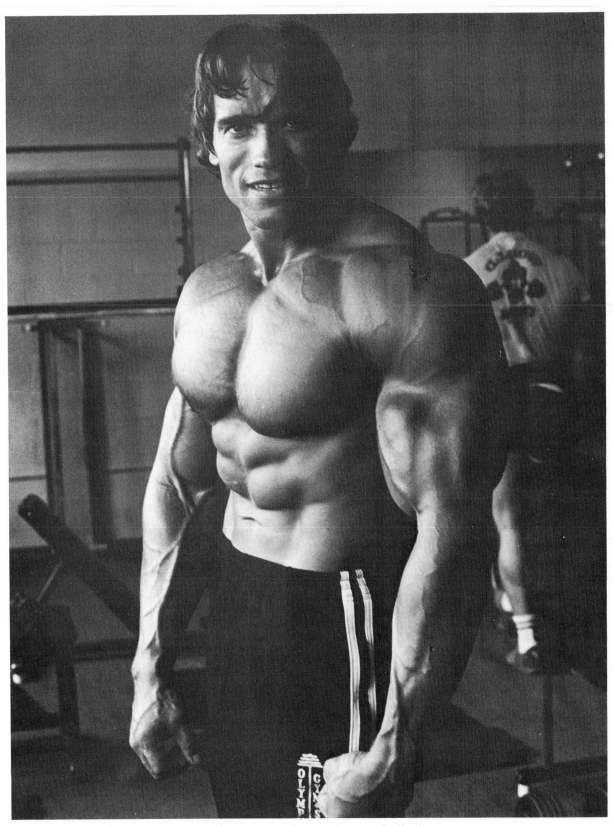

Arnold used his super genetics to build the world's most famous physique.

The Endomorph's Training

The endomorph needs to be motivated and kept enthusiastic, so he should surround himself with others when he is training. If he exercises in the company of others who are ultra-enthusiastic, that enthusiasm will rub off on the endomorph. If he opts to train by himself at home, chances are that he'll end up watching television and eating a bag of potato chips instead of hitting the weights.

A lot of endomorphs have a sluggish metabolism. Therefore, every exercise session should contain some form of really stimulating exercise to *step up* the metabolism: high reps, squats, running, rope jumping, and such like.

Extreme endomorphs may, in fact, be suffering from a hormone imbalance. All of us have hormones and some of the characteristics of the opposite sex, but a man who has wide hips, round buttocks, a rounded lower abdomen, little body hair, and noticeable fat on his pectorals might want to consult his doctor about the advisability of getting some hormone therapy.

Needless to say, the endomorph with his over-efficient digestive system must limit his overall caloric intake. He is, poor man, destined to be forever hungry. The food he eats should not be overcooked but as near to its natural state as possible. He should also avoid sugars, excess salts, and junk foods of all types like the plague.

Natural genetics helped Chris Dickerson to the top.

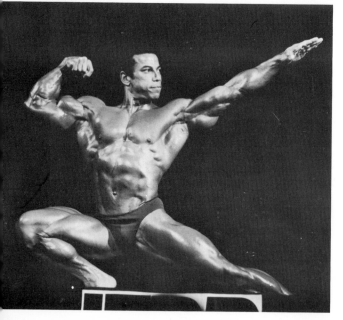

The Ectomorph's Training

Ectomorphs are slow gainers, with long, light bones, average muscularity potential, and poor ability to put on fat.

They usually read every article on gaining weight they can lay their hands on, and often their ambition exceeds their capacity. They embark on a schedule and keep adding "must" exercises to it until their routine has a horrendous length that takes hours to complete. They chop and change, change and chop. Some try a new schedule every few weeks.

Ectomorphs use up oceans of energy, never sit still, gobble their food, go to bed late, and are frequently tense and worried. No wonder they find it difficult to gain weight. An ectomorph's engines idle at double pace.

The primary needs of the thin man impatient to become a muscleman are to *slow down*, take life more steadily, and reduce worry and hurry to a minimum. It will be difficult for him. He must spend more time in bed, endeavor to relax after each meal (even ten minutes will help), and generally learn to relax more. Meals should be taken frequently, five or six small meals a day. Smoking and alcohol are definitely out, for they rev up the already high-revving nervous system.

More than anything, the ectomorph must tailor his routine to his wiry musculature. He will not gain on endless sets and reps. The routine must be severe enough to stimulate muscular growth, but brief enough to prevent nervous drain.

At the outset, eight exercises will be sufficient. Three sets of 8–10 repetitions. You may add an additional set and a couple of exercises as time goes on. Intensity, too, can be increased, but only in relation to your experience and condition.

Warning: Daily training is definitely not recommended for the ectomorph. Too much training is worse than too little. The ectomorph's secret is knowing when to stop.

The Mesomorph's Training

Lucky guy! I have known men richly endowed with very high mesomorphic components to gain without knowing how they did it. One man appeared to do it while ingesting little more than cigarettes and whisky. Another had

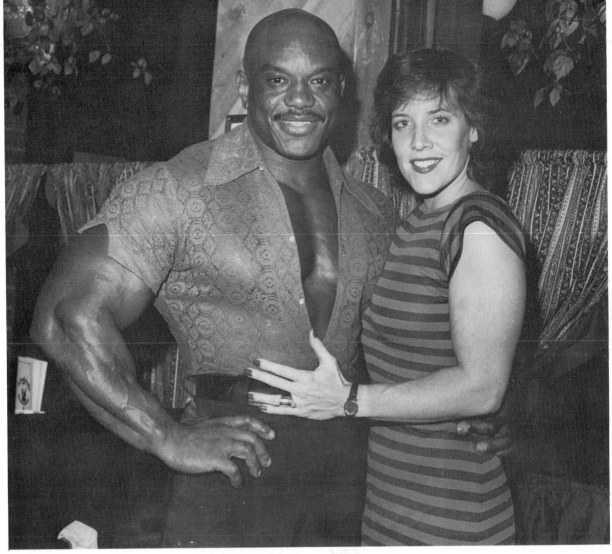

Sergio Oliva: When the gods created Sergio, they broke the mould.

no idea what he was doing. He simply trained on and off (more off than on), and much to the consternation of the regular, hard-training members of the gym, he grew and grew. A natural endowment of this kind may account for the poor training knowledge of some of our champion bodybuilders.

You yourself might know someone at the gym where you work out who may have been training for only a few months, yet has surpassed others who have been exercising for years. Could that man be a mesomorph?

It's more than likely. Mesomorphs often gain so easily that they give up training. Isn't that something? It's true.

I once knew a man who did nothing else but curl two 25 pound vinyl discs on a bar (total weight 70 pounds) once a week. He did no tri-

ceps work, no other exercise, nothing. His arms were just over nineteen inches. A mesomorph?

Another fellow, a truck driver, did no weight training, never did any at all. He was the laziest man I ever met. His arms are seventeen—cold. A mesomorph?

Yes, the mesomorphs are bodybuilding's Chosen People.

Of course, even the purest mesomorph will not make it to the top of the bodybuilding ladder just by his superior genetics. That may have been possible years ago, but today it takes more than mere heredity. There are so many variables: posing, diet, proportion, charisma—the list is endless. Today even the mesomorph has to train hard and use his head to get to the top. Incidentally, the most natural mesomorph I ever knew was Chet Yorton.

3
TRAINING LOG
The Silent Reminder

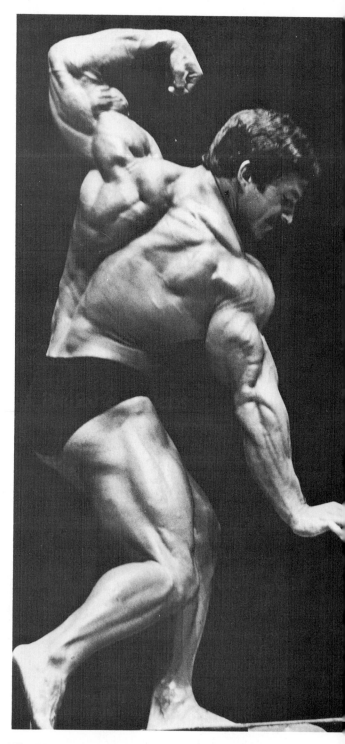

Record-breaking training is a must if body-building progress is to continue. Now that does *not* mean that you should constantly lift more and more weight at the expense of exercise style. Far from it. That is a fool's way of "progressing." You do, however, have to fatigue the muscles to a greater degree so that they rebel by overcompensating on a regular basis. Overcompensation means added mass.

Many bodybuilders keep a training log or diary to keep tabs on exactly what they have done in the past, and what they should aim for in the future.

Frank Zane, that triple Mr. Olympia, renowned for his physical shape and all-round perfection, has kept a training log since he first started training. Don't you wish you had done that? Can you really recall the exact weight, sets, and reps you were doing right at the beginning of your training?

Zane can go back up to twenty-five years with a few flicks of the pages! That's pretty handy information to have at one's fingertips! Not that Frank goes all-out each set every workout. He deliberately cycles his training with specific phases of work intensity. But even on a

Mike Mentzer records all his training progress in an exercise diary.

"down" cycle, Frank may attempt to break a record of some type.

The beauty of a training log is that it allows you to compete with yourself from one day to another, or one year to another. Imagine checking back to the same week last year to find that you were in fact doing ten reps with 300 pounds in the bench-press, when currently you can manage only four reps with the same weight! Now your training diary is, as Armand Tanny would put it, a silent alarm.

A log makes you pay attention to what you do and how you feel during a workout. It also brings a smile (or a frown) to your face when you look back over the years. The first thing you should write on the front page of your log is: *Ceiling Unlimited.*

One thing I know for sure: if you do not record your training details, then they will be lost forever. It's only the odd memories that you will be able to recall.

Always record every set (except warm-up sets) and every rep. Note the poundages used and also how the workout felt. Were you full of pep? Did a particular set seem easy, or did you feel drained during most of the workout?

When you achieve a new record in any exercise put a star (*) beside the set in question. Those stars will indicate your progress.

Record any injuries and the exact details of how they occurred. Were you trying a new exercise with too heavy a weight?

What about your food intake? This, too, should be recorded—not to the last morsel, but in its essentials. You should pay particular attention to recording whether you are supplementing your diet with vitamins, desiccated liver, proteins, minerals, etc. This way you will be able to check workout capability and efficiency against your nutritional intake. You will be able to gauge the usefulness of various nutritional supplements.

If the protein supplement you are taking is giving you constipation or diarrhea, say so. If you missed doing those all-important squats, record it. You goofed off and missed the workout altogether to go shopping with your girl friend? Leave a blank page.

Measurements, too, should be recorded. The tape measure doesn't mean everything, but if statistics are recorded along with your fat percentage, then you have some worthwhile data.

Lance Dreher: Mr. Universe.

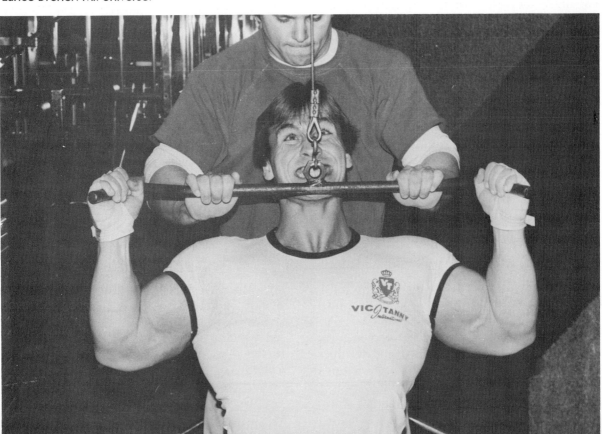

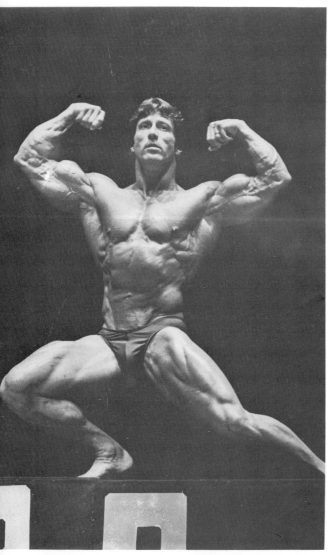

Frank Zane is noted for always keeping a training log.

Each day's entry must be dated. Note the time of day at which you train, your style of training (cheat or strict). If you are trying to shock a particular muscle into growth, then make sure that the details and the results are recorded. How are the muscles reacting? Do you get a good pump?

Remember that bodybuilding is not as it used to be. There are myriad different training principles. We are a long way from knowing all the techniques that can improve muscles. Routines, like records, are meant to be broken. With a training log, the continual upward adjustment will help you improve on a regular basis.

A training log will also help you pace your workouts. When you keep track of everything, you also become more aware that there is a tomorrow. You will be less inclined to go *crazy* for a *new* record at any particular session when you remember that you will have to do it again. Far better that your record book depict steady progress than a disorderly up and down. In other words, it is better to beat your previous "best" in small jumps rather than to go for large advances in weight progression that will make steady progress more difficult.

Also to be recorded in your log book are your training goals. Define your needs and wants. Write down your short-term goals (and your long-term dreams). When these things are in writing, they become much more valid.

The question may arise whether you should record your sets and reps at the conclusion of each set or at the end of the workout. This is entirely up to you. Some bodybuilders have no problem remembering their entire workout, while others have to write down the statistics at the conclusion of each set. The point to remember is that it must be done. Your concentration will not be ruined because you write down the number of reps you perform with a certain poundage after each set. Top bodybuilders like Mike Mentzer and Clarence Bass have kept extensive training logs and still trained with enormous zest, resting only a minimal amount of time between sets.

Most bodybuilders train in a free-style, unplanned, random manner, which is not conducive to progression. In order to reach maximum potential in bodybuilding, it is necessary to train in the most efficient and effective manner. A training log will help you maximize your efforts.

Whenever you have photographs taken, paste them into your log. Don't only include your best pictures. Sometimes the unflattering photos can help you more than a fluke shot that shows you looking like the uncrowned Mr. Olympia. After all, the training log is designed as a training aid, not as a showpiece for the rest of the world. Any time you find yourself putting in remarks that are untrue or merely wishful thinking, forget the idea! You are only writing yourself a valentine—a useless tribute to your ego.

A training log should record whether you are going to failure on your exercise, whether you are performing forced reps, negatives, etc.

4
MACHINES OR WEIGHTS?
Questioning the Superiority

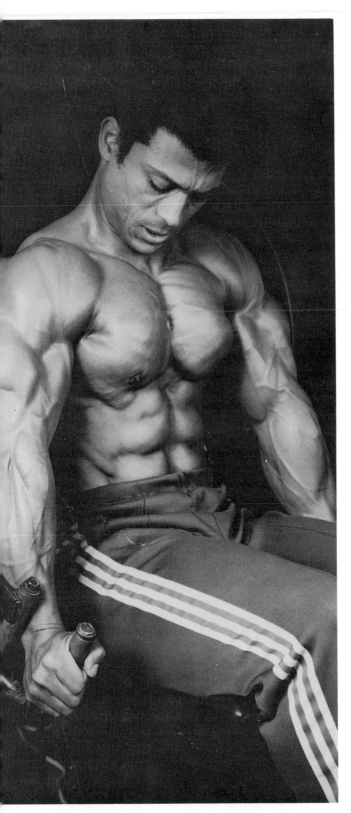

Mohamed Makkawy uses machines and free weights for maximum pump.

"Weights are for real men. Machines are for the sick." Are machines superior to free weights for building muscle? The debate rages on. One thing is sure: machines are getting more sophisticated all the time, and I suppose the time will come when machines will reign supreme.

Joe Weider has an interesting philosophy. He says: "I've had a theory for some time regarding a bodybuilder's aggressive nature, or lack of it. Most of the exercise facilities around the country today provide both machines and free weights. I have often felt that the more aggressive person would, if left to his own devices, gravitate towards weights instead of machines."

Ultimately, this theory was tested by Dr. Warren Chaney at the University of Houston.

A random selection of a hundred new gym members was divided into two groups of fifty. One group was given special instruction on exercises with machines only. The other group was instructed only in the use of free weights. None of these individuals had ever participated in a program of formal exercise.

Both groups then trained consistently for a month. One group used machines, the other used a variety of free weights. After that month, each group was cross-trained for a further month. That is, the free-weight users had to use machines, and the machine-trained people had to use free weights.

After those two months of exercise and indoctrination, the subjects were then "set free." They were told they could now structure their own programs and use any equipment they liked: either weights or machines, or a combination of both. Unknown to them, their choices were being recorded. Then Dr. Chaney matched the personality types with the equipment selected, and it turned out Joe Weider was right. The aggressive subjects selected the weights, while the unaggressive, almost without exception, chose to work only with the machines. It was also noted by Dr. Chaney that the individuals with the highest IQ's tended to choose a *combination* of weights and machines.

There is no doubt that machines play an important part in every modern bodybuilder's routine, but those machines are usually the old standbys. In rough order of popularity, these machines are: lat machine, thigh-extension and thigh-curl apparatus, and Hack machines. Those machines have all been around for twenty years or more.

There is absolutely no doubt that the regular squat has a greater effect on building size and strength in the thighs than any leg machine yet devised. Nor can one easily dispute that the wide grip chin is more demanding than its equivalent machine, the lat pull-down apparatus. But these machines do have their advantages. For example, the leg machines allow for multi-angle "attacks." There is no doubt that the Hack machine, the thigh-extension apparatus, and the leg-press machine do, in fact, "hit" the legs from a different angle. They do not challenge the "king squat," but they do have a value of their own, because they bring something unique to the angle, something that cannot be obtained from squatting. At present, this value is as an adjunct to free-weight training.

Getting back to the wide grip chin: it is the king of back exercises. At the least, it is on a par with the barbell row-movement. Wide-grip chins (behind neck) give you a "feel" that no machine can fully duplicate. But it is also true that the lat machine allows for a fuller range of motion, and one can certainly do more repetitions if one chooses to. Here again, a machine can bring something extra to a workout.

Ideal combinations, as we all know, often have us performing a few sets of free-weight squats, followed by a few sets of Hack machine exercises or thigh extensions. Likewise, chinning or rowing is frequently followed up with lighter lat machine work. (The angle of pull can be changed just by altering the position of your body in relation to the pulley.)

The proliferation of exercise machines on the market has been staggering. They employ a variety of devices, from heavy rubber bands, springs, redirectional pulleys, and cams, to air pressure, levers, and even water. Many have valuable uses, especially in conjunction with basic barbell and dumbbell movements.

When Arthur Jones first brought out his line of Nautilus equipment, the bodybuilders of the world got extremely excited. The propaganda for Nautilus (in *Iron Man* magazine in the late 1960's) was enormous, and I might add, convincing.

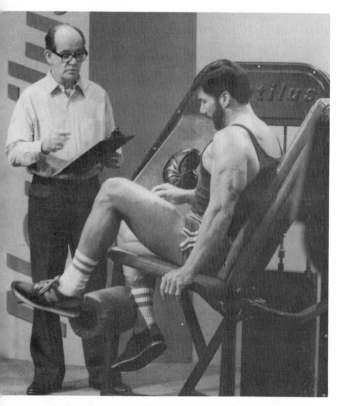

Arthur Jones, genius inventor of the famous Nautilus equipment, checks out physique star Boyer Coe during training.

When Arthur Jones writes, his passion comes through. He is one of the most inspiring writers on exercise that I have ever read. But Arthur made two mistakes:

1. He claimed that Nautilus training would produce top bodybuilders in a fraction of the time taken previously.

2. He attacked the modern disc-loading barbell as an obsolete, injury-causing antique.

Mistakes? The reported sales of Nautilus currently exceed $350 million a year, but as I write these words, Arthur Jones has not produced one single Mr. Universe or Mr. Olympia who built his physique exclusively with these Nautilus machines. Every one of them used barbells and dumbbells extensively. Nevertheless, it should be added that many Nautilus machines have some effects that cannot be duplicated by weights alone.

Further, it should be said that Arthur Jones is not finished yet. He is still pushing ahead with new machine ideas. The future will reveal what machine gems are in store for us.

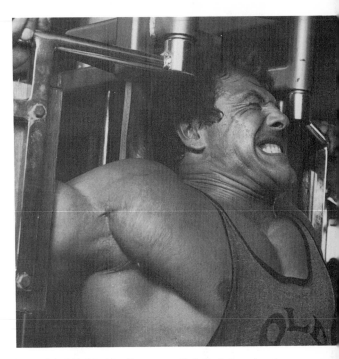

Canada's Reid Schindle uses a Pek-Dek for chest development.

As an example of the efficacy of machines, consider the following. For a long time a combination of bench-presses and flying exercises has been the proven way to big pecs. So you might ask, "What in heck did someone have to invent the Pek-Dek for?" Well, maybe Pek-Deks (Denie thought of that name) were not exactly *needed*, but there are several reasons to justify their existence.

1. Pek-Deks allow for a totally isolated pectoral movement, which means one can work the pectorals in an upright position without the added stress of exercising the triceps.

2. Pek-Deks are absolutely ideal for utilizing partner-assisted forced reps and "negatives," and they have none of the balancing problems associated with free weight.

3. Pek-Deks allow the "pre-exhaust principle" (that one is mine) to be used in a unique way.

4. Pek-Deks work the chest with less of an energy drain and in greater comfort.

So you see, the modest Pek-Dek has its uses. That doesn't displace the bench press as the chief builder of chests. But the Pek-Dek has a use, even if it is only used as added "variety." Remember the old "shock 'em" principle to maintain regular muscle growth? The Pek-Dek and many other machines do have specific uses.

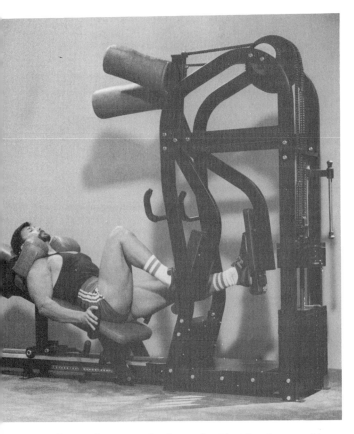

Boyer Coe goes for it on the Nautilus leg machine.

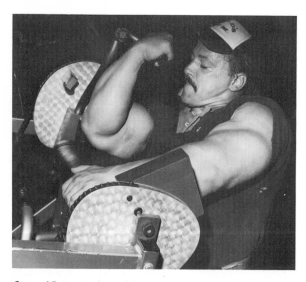

Casey Viator trains with Nautilus and free weights.

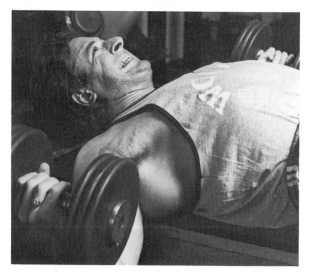

Greg DeFerro uses free weights in his workouts.

George Turner, the owner of the George Turner Gyms in St. Louis, Missouri, has some very interesting observations on free weights and machines. He is the first to admit that machines do have worth, and he has scores of machines in his various gyms.

"Forget the eye appeal," says Turner. "If the machine is not functional and valid, I will not have it!"

Mike Mentzer films brother Ray at the famous Nautilus headquarters in DeLand, Florida.

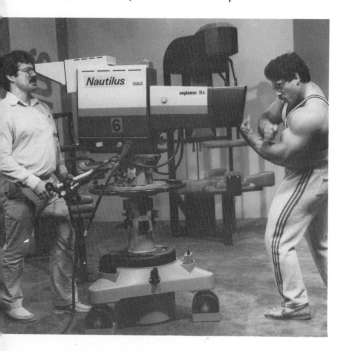

Writing in *Muscle and Fitness Magazine*, Turner points out that many salespeople and many advertisements make claims for machines that are just not acceptable to the experienced weight-training teacher.

"These machines invariably, even when the pivot points are set properly, as in the case with Nautilus equipment, which is adjustable for height as well, still do not, for the most part, take into account anything other than the height of the person. They don't consider other variables, such as length of the upper arm relative to the forearm, or length of the thigh relative to the lower leg. There are so many incipient variables like height and length and thickness of body parts, that there is no humanly possible way all these variables can be practically incorporated in the structure of the machine."

As an example, Turner cites the thigh-extension machine (cam, pulley, or weight type) where the pivot point is the knee. They are disadvantaged levers where the force of the lever required is displaced off of the joint. This is in contrast to the *natural* movement of the squat. "You pick up a heavy rock by squatting down and picking it up, not by hooking the top of your foot under it."

Squats build size—period. You cannot expect comparative size gains from using machines. Although the thigh extension has its uses, especially in patients recovering from cartilage surgery or in other knee-rehabilitation cases, it serves the bodybuilder too, but he must not expect great size gains from thigh extensions. It just doesn't happen that way. And the use of thigh extensions to failure is conducive to tendinitis, especially on machines where the movement starts when the lower leg is at an angle of less than 90 degrees. In fact, if any movement with the pivot point at a tendinous attachment is done to failure, it will invariably cause tendinitis.

Let's take the triceps. One of the most popular triceps movements known is the triceps pressdown on a lat machine. It is used by virtually ever top bodybuilder I know, and I can't think of one star who does not use it regularly. Yet, ironically, it is *not* a size builder. Granted it is a pleasant exercise, and it can sure rustle up a pump, but it does not help to stretch the tape at the end of the day.

Far better to use either the close-grip bench-press or the parallel-bar dip exercise (both work the belly of the triceps) than waste your time with Nautilus machine pressouts or pulley pressdowns.

You will also find that upright rows and overhead presses will do far more for your shoulders than cam or pulley-operated machines.

Nor will crossover cables and Pek-Deks give you the mass achievable with all forms of dumbbell and barbell bench presses and flyes. But as mentioned earlier, machines do have their uses.

I think machines will grow in variety and popularity, and I suspect many will achieve a degree of greatness. However, when it comes to building basic body mass, I can't imagine any machine, however well designed, that will better the basic, natural disc-loading barbell and dumbbell exercises.

What I think will (or should) happen in the sport of bodybuilding is that the inventors will get busy designing platforms and benches which will allow us to use an even greater variety of free-weight movements. We cannot change the straight-line one-directional resistance path of the barbell, because gravity pulls downwards only. But we can change the body position in a thousand and one ways, so that the barbell or dumbbell can work the muscles from different angles.

Free weights form the basis of a Barbarian workout. David and Peter Paul show how.

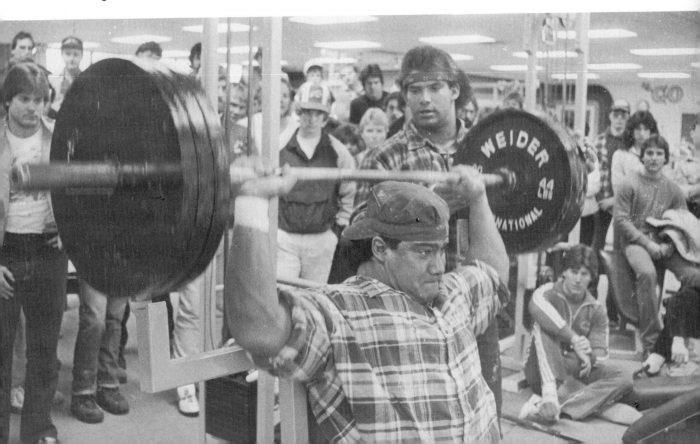

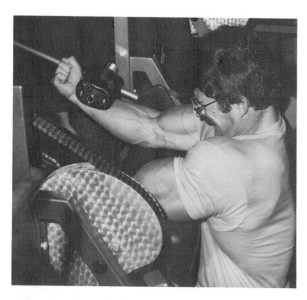

Mike Mentzer training on the Nautilus biceps machine.

One of the first units to do this was the flat bench, invented fifty years ago. This was a great development, believe it or not. Prior to that, the barbell men were pressing from a prone position on the floor. It wasn't until the forties that the incline bench came into use. Then we got moon benches, preacher benches, high flat benches, decline benches, and so on—all designed to change the angle while you are using free weights. Still there is room for more invention along these lines.

When the disc-loading barbell was invented, it was soon evident to the strength-and-fitness buffs of the world that this was a fantastic innovation. Almost overnight, it produced conspicuous changes in those who used it. Now everyone could look like a bodybuilder to a greater or lesser degree. Despite all claims, no machine ever made such an impact across the board. In fact, no machine or line of machines has positively been proven to build bigger muscles than free weights.

Mike Mentzer has made the point that although the vast majority of today's bodybuilders have trained on the free-weight system, their stand favoring free weights over machines is not entirely valid, since most of the bodybuilding failures, too, have used free weights.

According to Mentzer, free weights are not that different from machines. Furthermore, says Mentzer, "machines that work muscles which cannot be worked by a barbell are certainly justified."

With the Nautilus line, we got the first machine which tried to remedy the barbell's so-called disadvantage of only working the weakest part of a muscle (since only one part of the curl is difficult, but before and after that, it does not really tax the biceps). Since then, numerous other cam-operated machines have appeared on the market. The idea behind the cam, masterminded by Arthur Jones of Nautilus, is *to provide for automatically varying resistance that corresponds to the strength curve of the muscle through its full range of motion.*

When using a Nautilus, it is important to train in a slow, deliberate manner, so as to obviate any buildup of momentum. If you do try to "beat the clock" on a Nautilus, you will also be beating the idea behind the cam. In effect, the machine will become like a barbell, for you will find that your muscles will be taxed at one particular sticking point. Back to Square One!

I believe that all beginning bodybuilders should use barbells and dumbbells. That's the way to build a solid foundation. A novice will develop a feel for supporting and balancing free weights. He will enjoy the competitive aspect of lifting more and more weight. In addition, he'll benefit from using compound movements. Weights allow for more muscles to be brought into play (with the accompanying neuromuscular coordination) than machines. Most guided-resistance machines work the muscles in isolation. As a bodybuilder enters the intermediate stage, machines will play a part in his training—maybe an ever-increasing part. Machines can be used to hit certain parts specifically, and that can improve proportion, balance, and symmetry. Also, machines will often be very effective in conjunction with weights.

To sum up, let me advise you to forget the argument as to which is better, machines or free weights. (Remember when you had to like either the Beatles or the Rolling Stones?) Use the advantages each has to offer. At present, free weights are definitely the fastest aids to building muscle mass. Machines can help to etch in the quality. Of course, neither weights nor machines will be effective unless you work with them. Only total dedication and regular workouts will produce maximum results. And that's the bottom line.

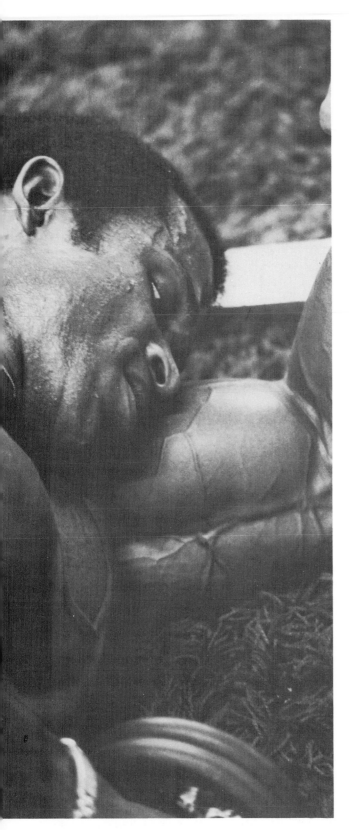

Serge Nubret, France.

5
THE REP UNDER SCRUTINY
Challenging Muscle Fibre Contraction

By definition, a "rep" (or repetition, to give its full name) means *more* than one. The rep is what bodybuilding is all about. It is the heart of your workout. As Mike Mentzer said (and does anyone say it better?): "The workout itself is the sum of all sets, but the individual rep is the basis upon which the whole is built."

For a long time now, the inventive minds of bodybuilders have been striving to maximize the effectiveness of the core repetitions that make up the bulk of our training.

Bodybuilders aspiring to added muscle size must understand that an individual muscle fibre (and there are millions of them in our bodies) either contracts *completely* or does not contract at all. They should therefore design their exercises so as to contract as many fibres as humanly possible in the course of a set.

The problem, then, is defined, and there is no shortage of strategies, plans, and principles devised to involve the thousands of fibres which go to make up the individual muscle groups.

Straight Set Reps

This is a basic system, still the most-used by beginners, intermediates, and advanced bodybuilders. It is the most effective and single most successful method of training known. A set is a series of repetitions (usually 6–12) which are performed continuously until the last rep is completed. More and more muscle fibres are involved with each repetition until the set is concluded. Even though the last repetition of a set is extremely hard, or even impossible, it is doubtful if anyone ever managed to stimulate 100 percent of the fibres in a particular muscle, as nature has not provided for such high levels of muscular exertion.

Most bodybuilders perform from 3–6 sets of an exercise when following this straight-sets system. However, total beginners are advised to perform just one set until they get used to the exercises.

Cheat Reps

The word *cheat* implies that you may be doing something wrong. In actual fact, the cheating principle (also known as "loose style") can be very useful if practiced correctly. Basically, one should not start to cheat during an exercise until the last rep possible in strict style has been performed. And then, of course, the less cheating, the better the effect. When cheating, one should never "snap" an exercise through its range; rather, use a gentle body motion to *aid* the muscles in getting the weight up.

Forced Reps

A training partner is needed for this method. When you are unable to complete a repetition using your own power, solicit the aid of your partner. He should then place his fingers under the bar and exert just enough pressure to let you make a lift you would otherwise fail with. More than two forced reps are not advocated.

Peak Contraction

A peak contraction exercise is one in which the muscle is under its greatest stress from the resistance (of a weight or a pulley apparatus) at the conclusion of a repetition.

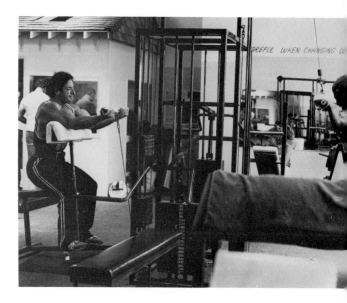

Rocky DeFerro and Roy Callender go at it at World's Gym.

The regular barbell curl is *not* a peak contraction exercise. The barbell passes through the most difficult part of the movement when the forearms are parallel to the floor, and there is definite relief as the bar approaches the shoulder area. The same type of relief is felt when one bench presses or squats. As the movement is concluded, there is very little resistance.

True peak contraction movements include wide grip chins, spider bench curls, wide grip rows, triceps kickbacks, standing leg curls, the crunch situp, gravity boot situps, and thigh extensions. Numerous machines also provide peak contraction exercises.

Actually, with some thought and rearranging of benches, pulleys, weights, and so forth, you can concoct dozens of new peak contraction movements. In fact, you don't even have to go that far. You can simply *stop* each repetition at the point at which you feel the most tension. (That is called a partial or half rep.)

Strict Reps

There is no doubt that ultra-strict reps have their place in a muscle-building routine. Few bodybuilders keep exclusively to strict form, but it is safe to say that most successful ones use strict repetitions . . . most of the time.

When you perform exercises in good strict exercise form, you eliminate the help gained by bouncing a barbell or swinging the body to get the weight up. In other words, you make the muscles themselves do all the work.

Starting the movement slowly is of prime importance when you exercise strictly. Do *not* kick out at a hundred miles per hour at the beginning of a leg extension. Start the lift at two miles per hour! Likewise, when you are curling a barbell or dumbbells, begin the lift slowly and deliberately. When you are pressing, begin methodically. No back bend or jerking! Never bounce out of a squat, for that will only work your butt and wreck your knees. No bouncing! When you are doing calf raises—also just deliberate up-and-down motions.

Rest-Pause Reps

This method has been used ever since barbells were invented. Rest-pause is not a system to be followed all the time, but it does permit you to make gains in tendon and muscle strength and in overall size in a few weeks.

It's a simple idea. After warming up for a particular exercise, you load up the barbell sufficiently to allow just one repetition. Assume you are bench pressing: press out one difficult rep and replace the bar on the stands. Let ten to twenty seconds elapse, and then perform another repetition. After a similarly brief rest, perform yet another rep—and so on. Each time you allow the body to partially recuperate. As the reps mount up, you may have to reduce the weight slightly to attain 6 or 8 reps.

Rest-pause owes its renewed popularity to Mike Mentzer, who uses it in his own rugged training program.

Nubret Pro-Rep Method

Serge Nubret of France has a unique way of training. At one time he trained very heavily and could curl over 240 pounds and bench press 500. Today he exercises using a singular, seldom-practiced principle. Nubret introduces progression into his training, not by constantly

Greg DeFerro has his wife give him extra resistance on the incline press.

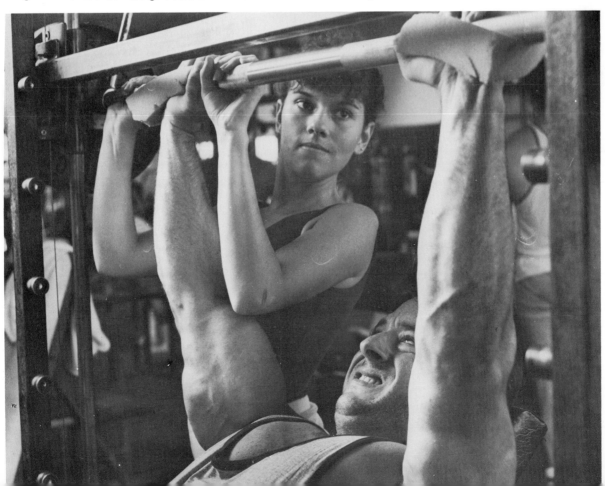

pushing the poundages higher and higher, but by pushing his rep count up. In actual fact it is a double progression, since he also tries to "race the clock."

If, for example, it took him 45 minutes to do 30 sets of an exercise one day, the next day Nubret will try to squeeze out 31 or 32 sets in the same length of time. He often wills himself to beat his rep record of the prior set. Using the seated dumbbell curl, Serge may start off by doing a set of 10 reps with a 45-pound dumbbell, and in his second set will do 11 reps, his third set 12 reps, and so on, all with the same weight. The secret of Nubret's method lies in his ability to "feel" an exercise by pure concentration on the movement he is doing at the time.

Superset Reps

All muscles are actually pulling muscles. They can only contract and shorten, and therefore they cannot push. The upper arm's biceps muscle, for instance, contracts and pulls the forearm upwards. The opposite movement (straightening the arm) involves the triceps muscles at the back of the arm, and they pull the arm straight. Even so, bodybuilders refer to *pulling* muscles and *pushing* muscles. Exercises under the *pushing* heading are the standing press, supine bench presses, pushups, triceps extensions, and leg presses. Often referred to as *pulling* exercises are upright rows, curls, chins, bent-over rowing, and thigh curls.

The original concept behind supersets was to alternate, rapidly and without rest, two exercises: one pulling, and one pushing. The most common combination was to alternate curls with triceps extensions. However, many champion bodybuilders would simply alternate two

curling movements or two pectoral movements or two triceps movements, not caring whether a particular muscle was worked alternately with its antagonistic partner (for example, the biceps and triceps).

Today the term superset merely indicates the alternating of two exercises in rapid succession. A few weeks on this type of exercising can jolt the muscles into new growth. It is a severe form of working the muscles. Too much of it could cause you to grow stale and bring you to a standstill. Paradoxically, a standstill can be broken with a week or two of supersetting.

Compound Training Reps

Compound training, sometimes known as "giant" sets, is definitely an advanced technique of muscle building. A compound set for the deltoids would involve doing three or four shoulder exercises, one after the other, with a minimum of rest between exercise. An entire shoulder routine using the compound-training principle could look something like the following:

Press Behind Neck	10 reps
Seated Dumbbell Presses	10 reps
Upright Rowing	10 reps
Standing Lateral Raise	10 reps
Short Rest	

Repeat the entire routine twice, for a total of three sets.

Pre-Exhaust Reps

I invented this technique around 1968, and documented my findings in *Iron Man* magazine in 1968. Pre-exhaust is the battering of a specific muscle with a carefully chosen isolation exercise, immediately followed by a combination movement. It is currently a great favorite with many top bodybuilders.

Let's use the chest as an example. As you may know, the triceps are involved in many of the recognized chest exercises, and in most people they are the weak link. That is, when you do dips, bench presses, or incline presses, the triceps are worked hard and the pectorals only moderately. This means that your triceps will grow more rapidly than your chest. That's fine if you already have a big chest; but if you want to develop your pecs, the best way is the pre-exhaust method. Here's how:

To get around the "weak link" triceps, iso-

No one puts in effort quite like Larry Scott. He trains to failure.

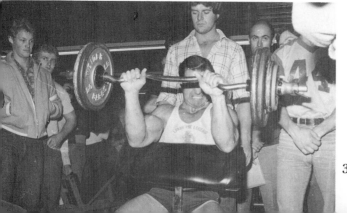

late the pecs first with an exercise like the dumbbell flyes, where the triceps are not directly involved. After a hard set, carrying the exercises to the point of failure, proceed immediately to the second exercise, such as incline or bench presses.

When you do the presses, the triceps will temporarily be stronger than the pectorals, which are in a state of near-exhaustion from the first isolation exercise. You are not limited by the weak link in the triceps.

Sample All-round Pre-Exhaust Schedule

SHOULDERS:
> *Isolation Movement:*
> Lateral Raise
>
> *Combination movement:*
> Press Behind Neck

CHEST
> *Isolation Movement:*
> Incline Flyes
>
> *Combination Movement:*
> Incline Bench Press

THIGHS
> *Isolation Movement:*
> Thigh Extension
>
> *Combination Movement:*
> Full Squat

BACK
> *Isolation Movement:*
> Chin Behind Neck
>
> *Combination Movement:*
> Bent-Over Rowing

BICEPS
> *Isolation Movement:*
> Scott Preacher Bench Curls
>
> *Combination Movement:*
> Narrow-Grip Chinning the Bar

TRICEPS
> *Isolation Movements:*
> Triceps Pressdowns
>
> *Combination Movement:*
> Narrow-Grip Triceps Bench Press

CALVES
> *Isolation Movement:*
> Standing Calf Raise
> *Combination Movement:*
> Rope Jumping

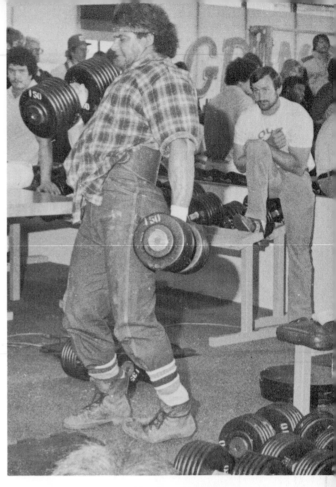

The strongest bodybuilders in the world? Barbarians curling with 150 pound dumbbells—totally unbelievable, until you see it!

Pyramid Training Reps

This method is very widely used because it allows the bodybuilder to start easily, build up to a peak, and taper off effectively.

Basically, you start with a set of high reps (12–15) to warm the muscles. In the following set, some weight is added and the reps are diminished. This is done with each set until only a few reps are possible. Then it is time to "come down" the other side of the pyramid. With each successive set, your weight load is decreased to allow for the extra repetitions. A typical pyramid routine for the bench press might look like this:

Set 1: 20 reps—120 lbs
Set 2: 10 reps—150 lbs
Set 3: 8 reps—170 lbs
Set 4: 6 reps—190 lbs
Set 5: 6 reps—210 lbs
Set 6: 3 reps—230 lbs
Set 7: 8 reps—140 lbs
Set 8: 12 reps—120 lbs

6
INJURIES
How to Avoid Them

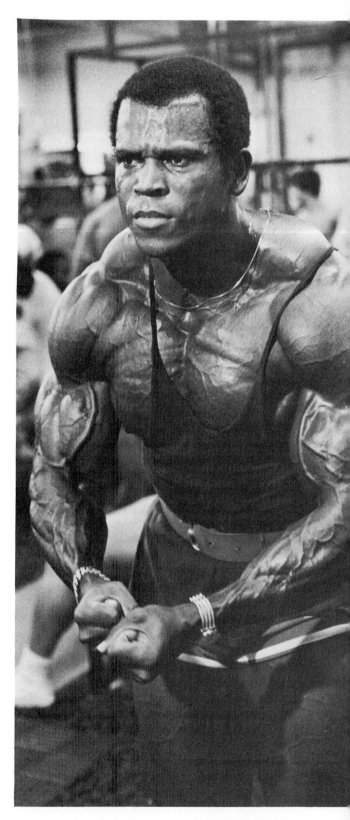

It is safe to say that virtually all athletes endure the constant risk of injury. The reason is, of course, that they keep pushing their bodies more and more, and unless things are brought along at the correct pace and in the right manner, injuries are almost inevitable.

The worst thing for a bodybuilder is not the pain of an injury (although that can be unsettling), but the annoying inconvenience of not being able to train as you would wish. Even a small muscle strain can keep you away from an all-important exercise for many months.

Weight trainers can incur injuries in the form of *tendinitis*, *muscle tears*, *strains*, *sprains*, or even *bursitis* or *hernias*.

The point I would like made very clear is that with common sense and care, there is no reason why you should not enjoy a successful bodybuilding career utterly and totally free of injury.

The biggest cause of injury to bodybuilders is probably carelessness, especially when trying to perform a near-limit lift. The show-off aspect to "having a go" is very conducive to sudden injury.

Serge Nubret always warms up his body before training. He has never had a bodybuilding injury.

Never be tempted to pick up a heavy dumbbell to heave it overhead. This can lead to a pinched nerve, which could cause you pain for years, with an almost immediate loss in muscle size in one arm.

Franco Columbu warns—and he should know, since he is a registered chiropractor—"Never begin your workout with barbell curls. The exercise itself is good, but do not *start* your training with this movement. Curls 'lock' the elbow joint, leaving the biceps vulnerable to injury."

Warming up is an integral part of training. Never neglect it. Before you go into any exercise, you should do at least one set of 10–15 repetitions with about 50 percent of your limit for that number of reps. If you do not like the idea of performing a high-rep warm-up, then do 2–3 sets of lower rep warm-ups, again using about 50 percent of your maximum.

Another way of inviting injury is to neglect the importance of keeping in the "groove." Let me explain. As we train, each of us develops a groove, or line, in which the weight travels. Take the bench press. The weight is invariably lowered to the nipple area of the chest. Year in, year out, you bench press in the same way. Your pecs build up. Your strength triples. But one day, while happily benching away with your regular poundage, you get the idea that maybe you should lower the weight to your upper pectoral. It seems an OK idea, so . . . wham . . . ouch! Something tears. Hot needles in your chest. You've done it: a muscle tear! Why? Because you put all the stress from the pectoralis major onto the pectoralis minor, an area that just couldn't cope with that kind of resistance.

When you get the idea that you want to change an angle or perform a new exercise, even if that change is minimal, you must approach it like a beginner. The bodybuilder who can bench press 300 must not change the groove. At least, not unless he's prepared to use only one-third of the weight. True, real strength will come quickly, but you can't force the issue without risking injury.

The same goes for any other change. You cannot suddenly do heavy incline presses if you have never done them before, even though you can bench press 500. If a new groove is to be forged, then begin with a light resistance and use a regular and unhurried progression.

You must take particular care in certain key exercises. The squat, for example: Always keep your back flat, head up, and lower slowly to the thigh-parallel-to-floor position. Never bounce out of a squat. Deadlifts should also be performed with a flat back, head up. Do not rebound the weight from the floor.

When performing bent-over rowing, keep your knees slightly bent, back flat. Actually, this is a deadly exercise, because the lower back is awfully susceptible to strain when you use very heavy weights. I would prefer you keep to T-bar rowing, or better still, single-arm dumbbell rows, where one arm can support your torso on a bench.

You wouldn't believe the number of bodybuilders who suffer shoulder tears. Because of their three-headed and complex formation, the deltoid muscles can easily become injured. Those injuries don't result from barbell presses,

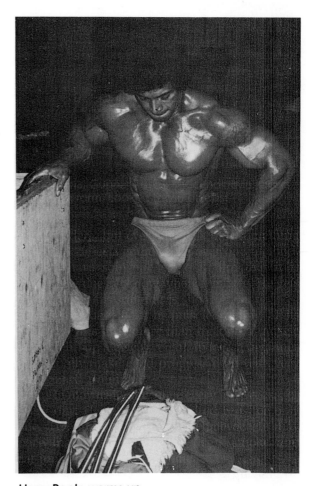

Harry Poole warms up.

35

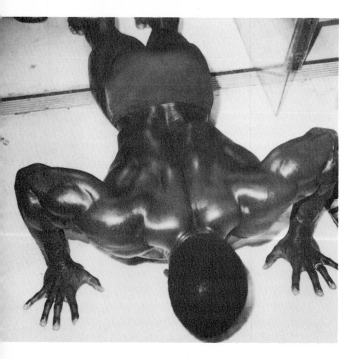

The most common warm-up exercise: floor dips. That unbelievable V-shape belongs to Tony Pearson.

builders as well as tennis players, wrist-wrestling champs, and house painters. Tendinitis can result from exercises which place a strategic joint in a vulnerable position. The single-arm triceps-stretch exercise, when performed with heavy weights, is an excellent producer of this painful condition.

It is sound policy to leave out any exercise which you suspect of causing joint or tendon problems. Either that, or limit the poundage

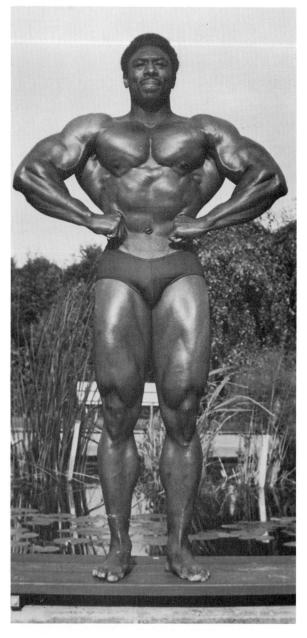

as often as from the precarious lateral raise movements. The reason behind this being that when you raise a dumbbell (elbows locked or almost locked) at arm's length, there are scores of grooves or pathways in which it can travel, and if you hit an unused groove with a weight that is too heavy, a tear may result—an unpleasant injury.

Another fiendish exercise, which correctly performed is little short of magnificent, is the preacher curl performed with either a barbell or dumbbells. The danger becomes magnified as the arms straighten, especially if the angle of the preacher top is shallow. *Never, never, never* allow the weight to bounce upwards from this straight arm position. Physique star Dave Spector did that, and it was Operation City for him as a result.

You should also beware of alternating certain exercises. One can alternate biceps and triceps exercises, for example, or chest and back. But particular care should be taken not to alternate chest and shoulder exercises. The muscle arrangement of these areas is likely to lead to unnecessary injury, if one is exercised after the other.

Tendinitis, the inflamation of a tendon, is another form of injury that can attack body-

Dave Johns, top pro bodybuilder, currently enjoying renewed success.

used in such cases. Take special care to concentrate on good exercise form. Good exercise style guards against injury.

Unquestionably, you are more prone to injury when your concentration lapses. So keep your mind on what your are doing. Do not listen to others while training. Pay attention only to what you are doing. The chatterboxes in the gym are wasting their own time. Don't let them waste yours as well.

What is pain? Pain is the body's defense mechanism warning you that injury is occurring or has occurred. The pain of lactic acid build-up in the muscle is acceptable as you push your reps to the limit. But sharp, searing, hot needle pain is different. It means a real injury is occurring, and you must immediately stop what you are doing. Try to determine the severity of the injury. Apply ice cubes directly over the area of pain as soon as possible. This will help to reduce the swelling and the inflammation. If the injury prevents you from moving your limbs in any direction, see your doctor. Competent professional help is always best, for even the smallest injuries can worsen, and in some cases they might become lifelong burdens.

Many bodybuilders who have injured themselves manage to "work around" the injury. That is to say, they continue to train but only use exercises that don't aggravate their condition. On no account should you perform any exercise that wakes up the painfulness of an injury.

In most cases, a torn muscle or strain or sprain needs rest. Subsequent training must therefore not involve the affected area until it has healed itself. Then, with great caution, resume regular training, always mindful of the *mistake* that caused the injury in the first place.

One helpful safeguard against injury, though no guarantee, is to practice some form of stretching exercise prior to beginning your workout. To get the fullest stretch, a muscle must be warm. Therefore in cold temperatures, a sweat-suit must be worn.

Flexibility is an important factor, and athletic coaches are recognizing that more and more. The proper method of performing a stretching program is to take your time and allow your muscle to lengthen gradually as you bend and reach (no bouncing or jerking). In all stretches in which you are trying for a maximum effort or bend, endeavor to hold the point of full extension for a full 15 seconds.

Preparation for Lower Body Stretching

Lean the body over as depicted in the forward position. Slowly . . . now. No bouncing. Hold the position for around 30 seconds, allowing your body weight to stretch the backs of your legs. You will feel some mild discomfort. As you get used to this attitude, it will benefit you to force it slightly. Try for a lower body position.

Bent Torso Pulls

As shown, lean over to one side and endeavor to pull the upper body down until the chest touches the thigh, using your arms. Keep feet at least a yard apart, and twist the waist into the direction that you are stretching without bending at the knee. Work each side 10 times and hold for about 10 seconds each time. This is an excellent movement for flexibility on the entire back, hamstrings, and calves.

Floor Stretches

Spread your legs outwards as far as you can. Working one leg at a time, stretch into the knee area with your head down. Try to pull your chest down to the thigh with the use of the arms. Hold the stretch for 10 seconds. Do 8 stretches to each leg.

Standing Groin Stretch

Standing with feet apart, pull down on each leg. If you wish to maximize the stretch, try to touch your head to your toes. Remember, no bouncing! Just slowly pull the body down to the toes and hold for 10 seconds. Try the exercise 6 times.

Back Stretch

Roll up on your shoulders, supporting the body with upper arms on the ground. Gradually and under control, lower your legs behind your head. Try to touch the knees to the floor by the sides of your head. Hold for 10–20 seconds, or longer when you get used to the position. This is very good for maintaining a limber spine, and you need only perform it once.

7
CYCLE
TRAINING
Pushing
to a
Peak

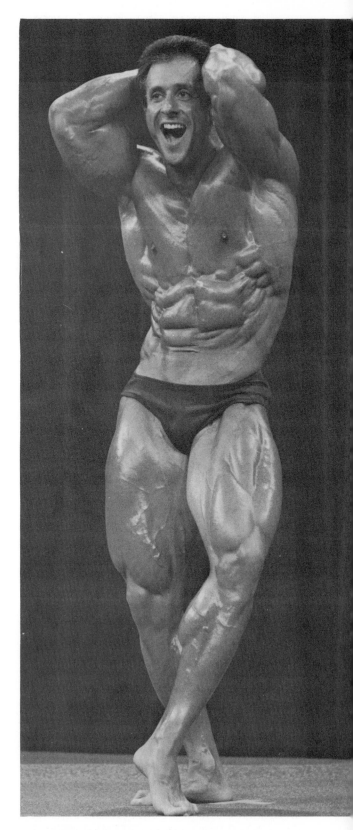

There's an old saying which you are sure to hate. In addition, you will hate me for even suggesting it. It has no place in a publication that is dedicated to musclebuilding—not fitting for a book entitled *Beef It!*

The saying? Ah, yes: *"Make haste slowly."*

The ironic thing is that if you push, push, push in your bodybuilding workouts each and every session, you will drive yourself into a sticking point.

There is a subtle difference between going all-out in your training *every* time and *cycling* your efforts to complement your physical and nervous systems. With cycling, you build up intensity to peak, and then you taper off and consolidate your gains by demanding somewhat less from your workouts. All athletes do this. It's a kind of controlled progress.

Any condition that you can maintain year-in and year-out is *not* a peak condition. Your body can be pushed to peak condition, but then it must rest. The edge will inevitably go, but it can be recalled and superseded with a new thrust. Making haste slowly applies very much to bodybuilding. In fact, it is the *fastest* way of building good quality muscle.

Rocky DeFerro—a great performer.

The philosopher Alfred North Whitehead said: "The only justification in the use of force is to reduce the amount of force necessary to be used."

I talked the point over with one of Canada's top amateur bodybuilders, John Cardillo. He is not totally enamoured with the idea of cycle training. After a lay-off, Cardillo likes to get back into shape quickly and drive at full speed, going all-out each workout. He feels that his body will tell him if he's overtraining, and that at such times he will rectify things by taking a few days off.

I am relating Cardillo's thoughts because there is a large number of bodybuilders who train in this way successfully. My own observation is that they are young and very enthusiastic and just do not burn out mentally.

Cycle training is usually practiced by the older or more experienced bodybuilder, who may not have an all-consuming, fanatical approach to his workouts. Day after day of blitzing his muscles just doesn't fit his temperament.

I would say that most, if not all, professional bodybuilders practice cycle training. Conversely, the majority of amateurs do not.

Clarence Bass, a great source of information, puts the case for cycling your training this way:

"Gains in muscular size and strength can only be forced temporarily. Long-term gains must be coaxed, induced in an agreeable manner, by gentle persuasion. Few bodybuilders are willing or able to strain to the limit continually. I doubt that anyone really wants to do curls, or any other exercise, until they are blue in the face—not on a regular basis, anyway. The mind rebels. It will not face such effort day after day. Bodybuilding progress, like progress in any other activity, is irregular; it's full of peaks, valleys, and plateaus. Don't expect to make continuous progress. A bodybuilder should push for a while, back off, and then push again."

One thing everyone seems to agree upon is that you can't run your body at full throttle *all* the time. You either have to cycle your training intensity or take occasional lay-offs.

Boyer Coe feels that layoffs are counterproductive physiologically. "You're much better off taking a period of what the Soviet weightlifters call 'active rest.' During this time, I do bodybuilding workouts of lesser intensity. I

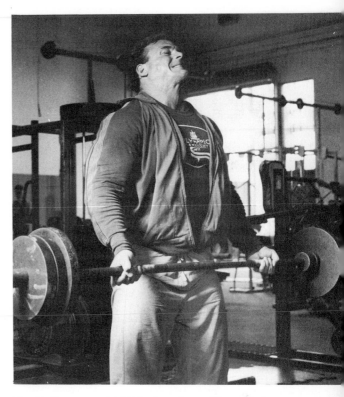

Tim Belknap, an AAU Mr. America with a great future.

also concentrate on building up my weakest body part."

Tom Platz has similar ideas. In the past he trained so hard that he sustained a mind-boggling list of injuries. In his eagerness to reach the top, he strained to a point where he injured his shoulder, tore his biceps muscle, brought on varying degrees of joint stress, and actually burst blood vessels in both his eyes. Mercifully, he has fully recovered from these injuries, and now trains with a good deal less intensity. "In the old days," he says, "I didn't know how much was *too* much. I have learned from my experience. No more torn muscles and burst blood vessels. Violent, massive, reckless effort is not the answer." Today Tom Platz trains more moderately, but he is still known as one of the world's hardest trainers.

Some bodybuilders cycle their training from one day to another. In other words, they perform a light (less intense) workout every once in a while. With some, this method involves two heavy workouts and two light workouts every seven or eight days. Others may choose to "go light" once every two weeks or so. The num-

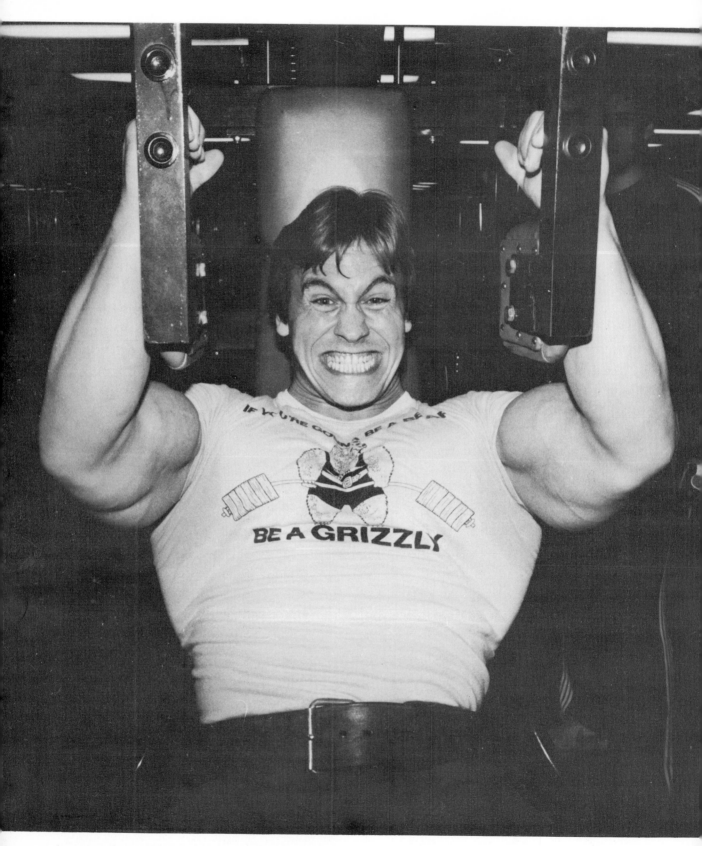

Awesome Lance Dreher cycles his training intensity.

ber of light (active rest) workouts you allot yourself will depend on your metabolism, your rate of recuperation, and your tolerance for vigorous exercise.

The most common form of cycling your training, however, is to gradually build up your training poundages, number of exercises, and duration of workouts to peak for a particular contest, and then to rest up by changing your exercise habits and down-grading your training intensity. Bodybuilders like Platz and Coe will stop all heavy training and increase their aerobic activities such as bike riding, running, swimming, all with one aim: to allow the body to regenerate. The comparative rest provides a sound base from which you can ultimately proceed to a new cycle of increasing intensity—for the next contest.

Cycle training is good for you. The body just cannot take a non-stop pounding, and that, as Vince Gironda says, "will bring on a state of 'overtonis'!" Even Mentzer believes in cycling his training efforts.

Also, there is evidence to show that those who push their muscles to failure and beyond for long periods of time and without interruption may overstimulate their adrenal glands, which then respond to the unrelenting stress by dumping excessive amounts of hormone into the bloodstream. It's nice to have a huge flow of adrenaline to help you in an emergency where you may have to run or fight for your life, but when this response is triggered too frequently, the adrenal glands become overtaxed and exhausted, with a resulting reduction in output. In short, you become lethargic, lose interest, and show all the signs of what is known as the "overtraining syndrome."

Research has shown that maximal stress cannot be endured for more than two or three weeks before this state of physical staleness sets in.

The answer, then, is to cycle your training to incorporate a steady, progressive build-up, but also to be aware of the dangers of exhausting the body's inner vitality. And when you plan on forcing yourself to a new plateau, do not make an all-out effort that exceeds two or three weeks. Chances are, you will be defeating your aims if you do.

After a contest or other event which you have peaked for, you will be better off if you

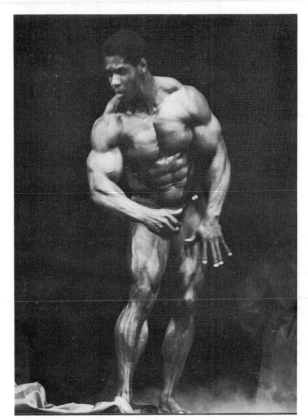

Bertil Fox—massive, even in repose.

wind down your training to a comfortable level with enjoyable exercises such as bike riding or sports. Do not pig out on food to the extent of getting fat. Make a point of not gaining more than 10–15 pounds over your competition weight. If you allow your body to bulk up too much, you only make things more difficult for yourself the next time around.

After your fun-and-games aerobic exercise, do not force yourself back into heavy training. Allow yourself time. Let the desire return to you naturally. It will come.

When the desire returns, harness your enthusiasm and control your workouts. You will be surprised how you can make your workouts steadily progressive even when you don't drive yourself with great intensity.

Ultimately, of course, when your next deadline (contest?) approaches, you will push for a new peak; and because you have held back and paced your progress, a new peak of development will *assuredly* arrive. Cycle training is used by all athletes. It works for them, and it will work for you.

8
POWER THINKING
Mental Programming for Success

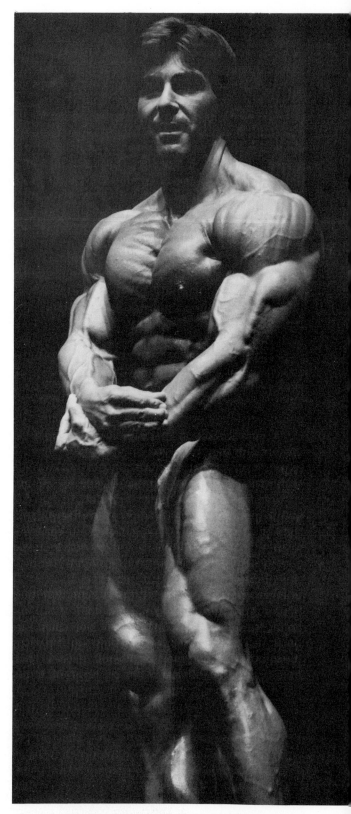

Dennis Tinerino (USA). He follows the principle of power thinking. What a sensational body!

Computers are with us for good. Like it or not, our bank has our financial status on computer and the government has our personal statistics on computer. They even have the audacity to give each of us a number—like a convicted criminal—and that number is on computer. Stores, credit card houses, libraries, licensing bureaus, tax offices, and who knows what other institutions, have information about every one of us on computer.

Rightly or wrongly, many of us resent the computer age and the invasion of privacy we suffer as a result.

Yet we, too, each possess a computer of our own: our brain. It is a relief to know that science has not even begun to approach the complex workings of this superstructure. Our brains are far more complex and versatile than any billion-dollar computer system invented by man.

The brain controls everything we do, or set out to do, and like a computer, it can be programmed. We can program our brain with aims, orders, and even enthusiasm.

Goals

The super-achievers in bodybuilding today have programmed their brains for success. They have set themselves on a path to physical achievement which, once set is not easily altered. They have set a definite goal. They are totally confident of their ability to achieve it, and they persist relentlessly in their quest.

Have you ever noticed that before you perform a set of repetitions as you lie down on the bench or take your hand spacing on the barbell—that you actually talk to yourself? This happens *every* single time, and there are no exceptions. Some bodybuilders even talk aloud. What is it they are saying? What do *you* say before you attempt a set?

The answer is that you tell yourself how much effort you are going to allocate to the movement. You program your computer: "I'll do 10 reps." "I'll try 6 strict reps, 2 or 3 cheating." "I'll go for 12 reps." If you didn't program yourself on the effort you need for a particular set of exercises, do you know how many reps you would do? None!

Goal setting, both for the short term and for the long term, is essential to success in bodybuilding. Listen to what Franco Columbu says: "When I'm not in training for a contest, I try to train heavy and hard. But my mind asks me why I am doing it if I am not getting ready to compete. So my body doesn't go all out."

Physical excellence contests on all levels—novice, state, national, international—serve to give bodybuilders the spark of enthusiasm that makes them train harder.

Always one to think things out, Arnold Schwarzenegger gives his friend Franco Columbu a pep talk before a heavy set of bench presses.

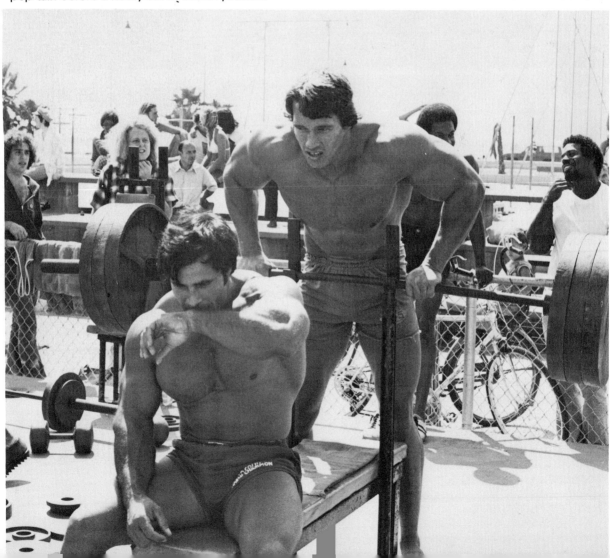

Mike Mentzer feels the same way as Franco: "During the greater part of the year, when no contest is imminent, my training is not fueled with the intensity or energy I know I am capable of generating. I operate well within my limits, failing, as William James might say, "to make full use of the powers I know I possess'."

Some bodybuilders, possibly most, do not have to program themselves in order to be full of enthusiasm or desire. They have an inborn quest for immortality. It comes naturally. They are driven like men possessed. They cannot stop training. Nothing else matters. They have caught the barbell bug. Tom Platz has certainly caught that bug. "Determination isn't enough to make a champion," says Tom. "To me it seems more like desperation. You can't just *want to*. You have to *have to*."

This is confirmed by bodybuilder and writer Denie, who says: "Some of the more successful bodybuilders are on the verge of being mentally disturbed individuals, such is their hunger and drive for success." Denie is the author of *Psychoblast*, a book which demonstrates how the mind controls and inspires the development of great strength and muscle size.

Visualization

It is one thing to believe in the power of the mind and quite another to harness that power. Visualization is one important technique for bringing the mind's power to bear on workout performance.

There is some evidence to show the way you visualize your performance before you actually attempt it will greatly influence the result. For example, if an Olympic lifter only half-believes that he can lift a certain weight, his chances of success are about 50 percent. If he has genuine doubts that he can lift a heavy barbell, then there is zero chance that he will achieve it. Conversely when you couple 100 percent of effort with 100 percent of belief in your ability to succeed, success will be achieved. That is the reality of the power of the mind. It is believed that visualization actually helps to develop the neural paths that are required for precise control of physical activity.

There is no doubt that incentives can so excite and inspire the mind that the effect spills over and produces a dramatic increase in physical effort and physical achievement. If your visualization or dream is vivid enough, the subconscious makes positive adjustments that clear the way and expedite the achievement of your goal.

Arnold Schwarzenegger wasn't the first bodybuilder to use visualization to help his muscles grow, but he was certainly one of the first to spell out exactly how he thought about his muscles when training. "When I am exercising my biceps," says the Austrian Oak, "I see them as two huge mountains, filling up the room, getting bigger and bigger."

Inspiration

Let's get back for a moment to Mike Mentzer's discovery of the writer William James. In his essay "The Energies of Man," James explains why some men are able to perform at a higher level than others: "Either some unusual stimulus fills them with emotional excitement, or some idea of necessity induces them to make the extra effort of will. *Excitement, ideas and efforts* are what carry us over the dam."

Boyer Coe relates how he uses music to excite his urge to achieve. "Sometimes when I go into the gym to train, I am anything but inspired to go at it hard, but as a lover of music, I get some of my heavy music going on the record player or radio, and my workouts quickly take on a new meaning."

Inspiration can come from sources other than music. Some bodybuilders find they do best by training with the opposite sex. In fact, numerous male bodybuilders make a point of selecting female training partners. This, they claim, provides them with the inspiration to bring their training efforts to a new high. Presumably, the women also derive inspiration from training alongside the men.

One famous bodybuilder who always has women as training partners admits: "When I train with women, no way am I going to fail with a particular weight! I have more incentive to give my everything to my workouts when I train with a woman. It seems to stir up my hormones, or flood my system with cholesterol, so that I double my efforts."

When you really believe in yourself, or are inspired by some outside force, and completely determined to achieve your goal, your mind releases the amount of energy you need to give it your best shot.

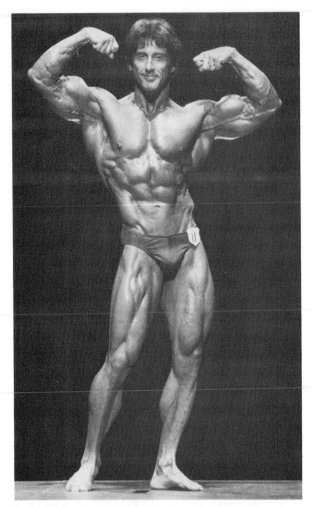

Frank Zane. He's long been famous for quality workouts and goal-setting.

Concentration

Concentration is one of the functions of the mind which has to be learned. It is necessary to give your total concentration to a particular set if you are to advance to a new plateau of physical development. But this is more difficult than you may imagine. Concentration means single-mindedness, holding one thing in your mind to the exclusion of everything else, and the mind has to be trained to achieve the ability to concentrate fully.

It has been said that the mind cannot easily concentrate on one thing for more than a few seconds, and if you can focus your attention on one thought or object for 12 seconds or more, then you have the ability to concentrate fully.

By using this type of focus on your sets, and by excluding all outside distractions, you will be using your mind to maximize your progress—and that is what you want, right?

Decide what you want from bodybuilding. Paint that picture in your mind, and follow through with the necessary action.

Ask any serious bodybuilder what got him interested in the sport. Chances are he will tell you that he saw a well-built guy somewhere, or else he saw a picture of a bodybuilder on a magazine cover. Either way, he was inspired to take up bodybuilding himself. Sometimes it is this first inspiration which is so powerful that it keeps the individual training madly for a lifetime. But in most cases the real stimulator that keeps a fellow training is the sight of his own progress. When you see your muscles growing; when you witness an increase in muscle strength, definition, and density; when friends start remarking about your development; . . . those are the times that the barbell bug truly bites into your ego and imbeds itself so deeply that you will never be rid of it.

Not that you would want to be. Having a healthy need for muscles and strength is a joy. Life has a reason for you. It is something to work for, an ambition to accomplish.

Sometimes, however, this muscle madness deserts us. It may be age, or perhaps some other interests that slowly have taken precedence. Nonetheless, you still want muscles. That concept never leaves; but sometimes the work one has to put in to achieve minimal results does not seem worth the effort.

It is at such times that we need to summon the power of our mind to program our brains for success. With enough mental effort, we can make ourselves into anything our genetic endowment permits.

Limitations develop as a result of limited thinking. Open the door to success! Seek to expand on what you already have!

Many potentially great physiques are held back by lack of positive programming. You can meet a guy with enormous Mr. Universe potential, only to find that mentally he will never pull it off. He does not believe in himself because he is full of negative programming.

You can train your mind as hard as your body, and in so doing, totally control your bodybuilding gains. Bring your muscular development to what you want it to be. Develop confidence, poise, and charisma, and come out a winner.

9
SUPER-STRUCTURING YOUR ROUTINE
Improving Your Level of Efficiency

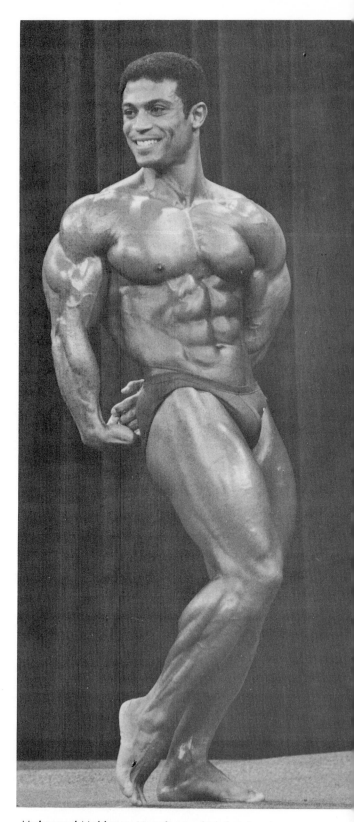

Mohamed Makkawy transformed his body when he superstructured his physique.

Most of my day is spent indirectly working on my magazine, *MuscleMag International*. I am on the phone to writers, photographers, and bodybuilders for about 30 percent of my time. Another 30 percent is spent on organizing articles, photographs, and artwork that will or will not appear in the magazine, and on correspondence with my contributors.

But a whopping 40 percent of my day is spent in my Muscle Store in Bramalea, Ontario (the address is Unit 7, 2 Melanie Dr.), and there, much of my time is taken up by discussion. You can guess what the topic is. It's bodybuilding. More specifically, how to make the fastest progress possible.

Now, I myself have been in this game for thirty years. I have written scores of courses, dozens of books, including *Hardcore Bodybuilding* which actually made the best seller lists. I started *MuscleMag International* from nothing and built it to its current position of being the second biggest seller of all the bodybuilding magazines on earth! I also invented the much-used "pre-exhaust" technique.

Big deal! I'm still a schmuckkkk! Why? Because I still can't tell *you* exactly how to train. All my experience, I often think, has taught me only this one thing: that *there is more than one way to skin a cat!*

Every summer literally thousands of aspiring young bodybuilders make the trip from all over the States and Canada, some even from Europe and Asia and Africa, to the mecca of bodybuilding: Southern California. In their hordes they visit Gold's and World's gyms in Venice, a suburb of Los Angeles, or Vince's Gym in North Hollywood. Many have saved all year to make the pilgrimage of six, eight, ten weeks, what have you; and they've all got the same purpose: to learn from the stars, to be in their proximity and get the real dope on training. As Vince Gironda says, "There are more books, magazines, and training establishments than ever before in the history of bodybuilding; yet everybody is looking for one thing: information. And they can't get enough of it."

When these keen young bodybuilders get to California, they are subjected first to shock and then to confusion. Here's how it works. When they finally find Robby Robinson, or Tom Platz, or one of the thirty stars they have come to see training, they are shocked out of their socks because they see their favorite superstars using standard barbell and dumbbell exercises. Somehow, they expected to see something new and secret being performed, but no, sir! Robby is over there doing barbell rowing. Greg DeFerro is doing calf raises. Franco and Arnold are doing barbell curls. Lou Ferrigno is bench pressing, and Platz is squatting. Our budding bodybuilder can't believe his eyes. It's all so *normal* that it is *shocking.*

Ironically, in spite of all this normalcy, our muscle pilgrim is beset by *confusion*, because after a few weeks he is confronted with so many permutations of how often to train, how many sets and reps to use, what food supplements to eat, how much weight and intensity to use, that he just doesn't know where he is with his own training. Chances are, if he asks six bodybuilders for the best way to train, he will be given six different answers. Thus confidence and hope turn into confusion and despair. Our traveling enthusiast came to the mecca of musclebuilding to learn the most advanced training techniques from some of the world's top

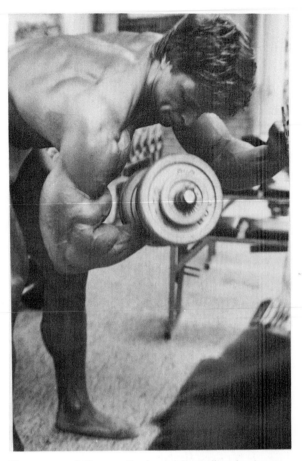

Phenomenal Gunnar Rosbo of Scandinavia shows his curling form. Look at those biceps!

bodybuilders, but everyone tells him something different. He gets enthusiastic over one method, only to have someone else tell him that it is wrong. He doesn't know what to believe. He gets so confused, his training is shot to hell.

When one looks at musclebuilding at its *simplest*, it is little more than making a muscle work to lift up a given weight. In fact, a beginner can usually make good progress even with very haphazard training.

He may train only once every few weeks, or every day. He may do a hundred reps, or only one. Twenty sets, five, one—whatever. He may party instead of sleep; he may drink, smoke, and eat junk, but gains will come.

Yes, it does happen. It shouldn't, but it does. So much for scientific bodybuilding.

But when you break all the rules, you'll pay for it sooner or later. Your early progress will not continue because of one unalterable fact: *The bigger you get, the harder it is to get any bigger.*

O.K. So in the beginning even totally inefficient training will give results, but in time the gains will slow down or even come to a halt. It is at this time, whether your prior training methods and habits were merely inefficient or downright abysmal, that you will have to take stock of yourself. From now on, you must maximize your workout efficiency. That means each variable must be given attention. In short, you must do your best on all fronts.

Apart from your diet, food supplementation and relaxation, there are numerous variables involved in your training. They are: number of repetitions, number of sets, speed of training, order in which exercises are performed, amount of weight, number of workouts per week, amount of rest between sets, choice of equipment, number of exercises used, strict or loose exercise style, positive or negative mental attitude to your training.

Right now, it is an odds-on bet that your training, in its myriad of variables, is not as efficient as it could be. It's only a guess on my part, of course, but you could probably improve the quality, the efficiency, and the workability of your training schedule a great deal.

Training Intensity

To keep a muscle growing, you have to keep increasing the punishment you are delivering the muscle on a regular basis. This very fact is enough reason for *holding back* in your workouts. Let's assume that you have just enjoyed a break from training because of holidays, school exams, job, or what have you. Well, it would hardly make sense to jump right back into huge all-out super strain workouts, would it? No, sir! You would probably end up with sore and injured muscles. The correct way to go about getting back to training is to make a slow but planned effort to pace your training intensity and workload progressively.

Progression

Only do today what you can supersede tomorrow. Far better to increase your bench press by five pounds this week, knowing that you can add another five pounds the next week and another five pounds the week after that, than to go all out now and fail progress later on.

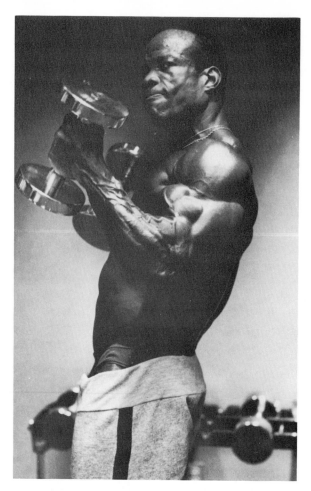

Al Beckles performs the standing dumbbell curls at the Playboy gym in Atlantic City.

You see, once you have lifted a weight heavy enough to stimulate your muscle fibres, lifting a heavier weight doesn't give you better results. That's why, when you go to Gold's or World's gyms, you will often see a champion bodybuilder using. only light or moderate weights. He is at the low end of a cycle and is beginning to increase intensity on a regular basis. Each workout he will do a little more. Perhaps he'll add another set, or maybe he'll add a few pounds to the bar. The important thing is that if he is only handling 40-pound dumbbells, then that is all he needs at this time to stimulate growth. As he nears the time of a competition, he may well be using 60-pound dumbbells, but he will not have made the transition with just one or two jumps. The poundages, reps, and sets will have to be progressively earned, one small step at a time.

How Many Repetitions?

Theoretically, one could justify the single (all-out effort) rep system for building the largest muscle size. Some weightlifters are after explosive strength and use that system. But such a system does not serve the bodybuilder's needs. The competitive weightlifter, who attempts to fire off as much muscle fibre as possible within the few seconds it takes to complete a single rep, will not gain the overabundance of muscle tissue that the top bodybuilders strive for. For muscle-building purposes it is far better to use a lower percentage of muscle fibres each repetition, but with a higher overall count. In this way the nervous system is forced to recruit as many additional muscle fibres as possible. You need to fatigue the fibres with repetitions, overloading your muscles regularly with repeated sets of 8–12 reps, progressively overloaded (moderately increasing weight resistance whenever possible). This will give you the kind of body development you've always wanted.

Triceps pressdowns, Barbarian style.

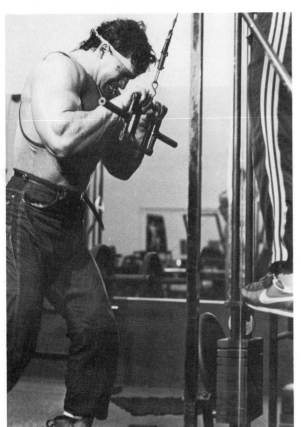

Volume is important, since it serves two purposes. It contributes to plumping up your muscles cells individually, and it helps you to build new capillaries (which come as a result of regularly performing plenty of sets and reps).

This is why trained bodybuilders get a much bigger pump than Olympic lifters. Most advanced bodybuilders can add well over an inch to their arms by doing a few dozen close-hand floor dips.

Another fact that has come to light and is the result of volume training is that the glycogen stored in the muscle can be greatly increased. According to bodybuilding author Bill Dobbins whose knowledge I greatly admire, "Glycogen is carbohydrate energy stored in the muscles. For each gram of glycogen, the body will store 2.7 grams of water, all of which adds to muscle size and shape." This is why glycogen-starved bodybuilders who are on too low a carbohydrate diet appear stringy and small. It also explains the usefulness of "carbing up" the day before an important contest (usually done by eating a plate of spaghetti or a baked potato).

Having given you the case for a workout consisting of plenty of sets and reps, now let me say there is also a case to be made for power-building techniques (as used to prepare for powerlifting) on an occasional basis. Using heavy weights for lower repetitions cannot only act as a tonic, but can give the muscles a new dimension of experience. (A change is as good as a rest.) Franco Columbu, Frank Zane, and hundreds of other bodybuilders do occasionally employ heavy training. It improves the strength of muscles, tendons, and ligaments, among other things, and that is useful for achieving higher repetitions and upgrading training poundages when more regular workouts are resumed.

Exercise Style

Watch Roy Callender train. His curls are magic. There is a rhythmic flow, a cadence that is beautiful to behold. For the most part, you should train with good exercise style, working your muscles over the fullest range possible. For instance, start your curls with straight arms; do not start with torso leaning forward, elbows bent, swinging the bar up.

Cheating (loose training style) is a very so-

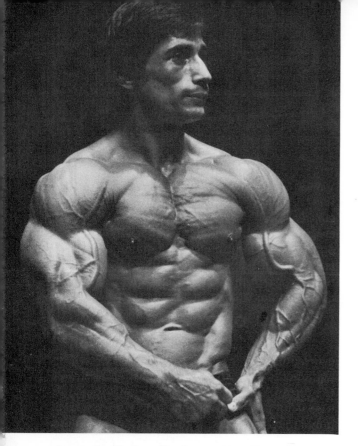

Danny Padilla from Rochester, New York.

phisticated technique. You need to know *how much* to cheat, and more importantly, *when*. Arnold Schwarzenegger made a habit of training in a very strict style for the first eight reps, and then he would cheat more and more as he labored through the last four reps. That way he got the benefit of both styles, but only after he had exhausted the benefits of doing eight quality repetitions in faultless exercise style.

Speed of Training

Increasing the speed of your training (reducing the rest time between sets) is another form of increasing intensity. But again, one must use the method intelligently. Make your rest periods progressively (that word again) shorter as competition or peaking date closes in. Naturally, more rest would be needed between sets of squats than between sets of curls.

Number of Workouts per Week

Do not base your workouts on a 7-day schedule. Your schedule should be dictated by your body's needs, not by tradition or custom. Of course, your schedule must also take your job or

school situation into account, but if you train at a gym that does not remain open on the days you want to train, then change to one that does!

Since muscle that is worked hard takes a considerable time to recover fully, you should not train the same body parts every day. Training frequency, like schedules, sets, reps, and intensity will and *must* vary with your training aims, and recovery ability.

One of the most workable systems for adding muscle size is the every-other-day split. For the benefit of the uninitiated, the every-other-day split involves splitting your workout schedule roughly in half. Perform the first half on one day, and then rest completely (no training) the following day. The day after that, perform the second half of your routine. The following day, rest from all training. In other words, you do half your routine every other day, and you never work out two days in a row. Mike Mentzer made his best gains ever (for the 1980 Mr. Olympia) by this method.

Increasing the duration, intensity, and frequency of your workout will ultimately arrive at a sticking point. The every-other-day split may be for you.

Canada's Reid Schindle gives everything to his incline flyes.

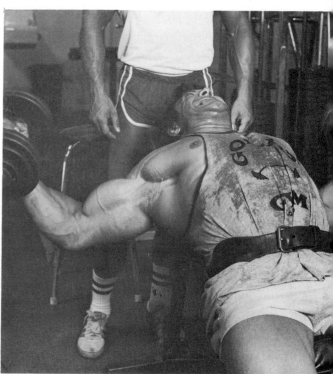

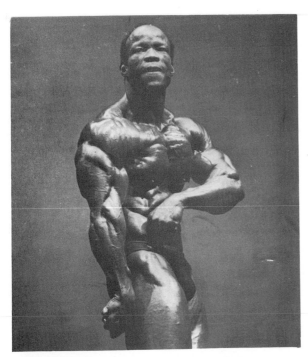

Albert Beckles. A super example of modern training methods.

Number of Exercises

Your routine must be built from need. You may want to do two or three exercises for a stubborn body part but only one "carry along" exercise for an easy growing area. At the *least*, the number of exercises you slot into your routine must be adequate to serve your basic growth needs. At *most*, they must stimulate growth without leading to staleness.

Amount of Weight

In a sense the weight you use in an exercise is totally irrelevant. After all, your muscles can't "see" whether you are holding a 20-pound dumbbell or a 50-pounder. Some "cheat artists" can bounce-hoist huge poundages, yet couldn't lift half the weight if they used the correct, strict exercise style.

Read the following carefully, it is true: *One important difference between the bodybuilder who wins titles and the one who tries but fails is that the pro uses barbells as tools for gaining muscle, not as weights that have to be heaved up.*

Choice of Equipment

There are not enough machines to take care of a bodybuilder's needs. You have to use free weights (barbells, dumbbells, and pulleys), if only for the needed variety. It just so happens that free weights are terrific for maximizing muscle size.

Bear in mind, too, that most bodybuilders do use some machines to supplement their weight workouts. Variety is the spice of life (and bodybuilding success).

Order of Exercises

It is not a good idea to perform exercises randomly. Group body parts together so that one area is fully pumped before moving on to another area. Perform heavy (demanding) exercises early on in the routine while you are full of energy.

Always scientific—the training of Serge Nubret.

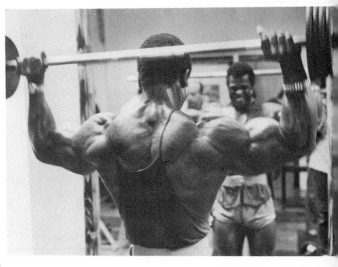

Training Attitude

Your mental attitude must never be less than 100 percent positive. Your success strategy must, unfortunately, incorporate selfishness. Relatives, friends, spouses, and lovers must come to understand that workouts are something that you simply must not miss. It may be difficult for them to understand, but that's the championship path. In addition, you must learn to see yourself as a bodybuilding success. (You just haven't collected your trophies yet.) You must maintain your positive attitude in every rep of every set of every workout. Concentrate on every exercise with all the dedication you can muster!

10
RECUPERATION
Mending the Muscle

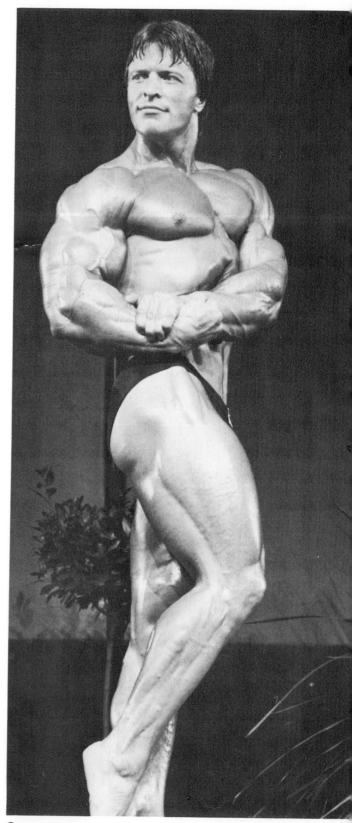

Gunnar Rosbo, Swedish giant.

Mike Mentzer, that bastion of sensibility, said it simply and best: "Any amount of training—whether it be short or long—is always a negative factor, in that it drains some of our resources. The less we disturb our recovery ability, the more we will have available for growth."

Recuperation is vital for the bodybuilder. The faster he recovers from a workout, the sooner he can train again. And the sooner he can train, the faster he will grow. On the other hand, if recovery from training does not materialize, then further training cannot give a positive effect. In fact, just the opposite can occur. You will grow stale and lose size, strength, and even enthusiasm.

Repeated training without *full* recuperation will dig you into the deepest sticking point ever. Your motivation will suffer; your muscles will shrink; brute power will ebb; and—hell of all hells—the pump will evade you. Gironda has a word for it, his own word: *overtonis*. Hear his pronouncement:

"Overtonis is my expression for the condition caused by too many sets and too many different exercise combinations, for the overwork which causes muscle tissue loss, hormone depletion, weakness, a smoothed-out or stringy appearance, inability to produce a pumping effect, and general lassitude or weakness. Overtonis stops the central nervous system from pumping blood into capillaries that might otherwise rupture. It is a safety valve activated by hormone loss. Going past the pump (too many sets when the body is not used to it) is the most common cause of overtonis."

Poor recuperation first rears its ugly head the morning after. That is to say, the day after your workout. As you open your eyes to a new dawn, you feel decidedly groggy. In fact, you may feel disinclined to get out of bed. You feel tired and lack interest generally. Your body is saying to you: "Boy, I *really* had a workout yesterday. I need more time to recover."

This tired, almost exhausted feeling you have on arising is not always accompanied by sore or aching muscles. What sore muscles usually mean (but not always) is that the body is recuperating, and that the healing process is well underway. Of course, if there is any soreness present, the muscle has *not* fully recuperated, but at least the healing process is taking place. The general opinion is that a *slight* soreness in the muscle the next day is ideal. It shows that your workout routine *got* to the body. But if the soreness is extreme, then you have overdone it, and adequate recuperation will take longer.

Workouts

One of the tricks of hastening recuperation is to not surprise your muscles too vigorously. There is a fine line between stimulating your muscles with new exercises, more intensity, and added sets—all for the sake of keeping them growing—and the obvious mistake of going all out with these tactics and reducing the likelihood of adequate recovery.

Let's take an example. Imagine you have always done 6 sets of 15 reps with your calf work, and you decide that you need to jolt your lower legs into growth by trying something new. Well, you could add on three sets of donkey calf raises. That would give the calves a *new* exercise, and you would also be making the overall calf work routine longer (more sets). But suppose you wanted to give those calves a *real* surprise. How about suddenly doing the new donkey raise movement for 20 sets? Wouldn't that be better? Would such a change not shock them into growth? The answer, of course, is No! You would be lucky to walk the next day—let alone boast additional lower leg size—and you would probably not be able to train your calves again for a week or more!

Let's get back to Mentzer. The high-intensity, low-set exercise he advocates will definitely hasten recuperation. Once the body has become used to this method, your recovery from workouts will be brisk. Mentzer said: "When I was using 10 sets for every exercise I felt constantly tired. Progress was slow. Now, with my heavy-duty program, I recover very quickly after workouts."

Still under debate, of course, is whether full intensity workouts are right for everybody. Does everyone gain from these heavy-duty workouts? Chris Dickerson, Mr. Olympia '82, is one of the many champions who does not agree with training to failure. Joseph Miller, a sports medicine authority, wrote the following in *Muscle and Fitness Magazine*:

"Physiological research indicates that the adrenal glands can become thoroughly oversaturated and exhausted if they are forced to overcome maximal stress for any period longer than 2–3 weeks. If high intensity effort is sustained beyond this time, the adrenals will be forced into total remission, and training efforts at that point will illustrate this."

The knack, of course, is to train the body without fatiguing it beyond its power of swift recovery. If you do not "heal" between workouts, you will not grow. The possibility of overtraining looms ever present with the competitive bodybuilder (especially when doing leg work), so we must perform the minimum amount of exercise that will stimulate continued muscle growth. Doing more sets than are necessary to induce growth will only hold back the recuperative process.

Peary Rader, the publisher of *Iron Man* magazine, has spent almost forty years advocating "abbreviated" training programs. The reason? To effect better recuperation. Following a workout the body must recover and replenish what was used up during the workout. It is only after full recovery has taken place that growth can occur.

If you use high intensity (forced reps, negatives, etc.), then you will be fatiguing your body to a greater degree. This increased intensity causes your body to produce increased amounts of lactic acid—hence the greater fatigue. Therefore, when you adopt a more severe program, slide into it by steps. If you increase the volume and intensity of your workouts gradually, your recuperation will likely keep pace. There is no doubt that a body which is coaxed into handling more will also "learn" to recuperate more quickly. It adapts by becoming less fatigued as your workouts continue. In short, the bodybuilder who keeps to his training and follows sensible health rules will develop the art of fast and efficient recuperation—within limits, of course.

Overtraining

Overtraining has additional hazards. It weakens the body's resistance to infection, making you more susceptible to the common cold and to flu bugs and germs that could lay you low for a week or more. Writing in *The Sports Medicine Book*, Dr. Gabe Mirkin lists the following signs of overtraining.

Muscle Symptoms
Persistent soreness or stiffness in joints and tendons
Heavy-leggedness

Emotional Symptoms
Loss of interest in training
Nervousness
Depression
"I don't care" attitude
Inability to relax
Decreased academic work or performance

Warning Signs
Headache
Loss of appetite
Fatigue and sluggishness
Loss of weight and muscle size
Swollen lymph nodes in neck, groin, or armpit
Constipation or diarrhea

Mike Mentzer describes a simple method by which bodybuilders can check on their condition: "For decades one of the most popular methods used to detect overtraining was to monitor the morning pulse rate. Upon rising, the athlete would measure his pulse for 60 seconds. If it was 7 beats a minute faster than usual, a layoff or reduction in training was indicated."

There are more sophisticated ways of measuring fatigue toxins in order to determine whether you are in an overtrained state. One way is to measure the enzyme levels in the blood, since damaged muscles release more of these proteins. Sports doctors who monitor their athletes carefully know that when the enzymes exceed a certain level, the athlete has to slow down.

Actually, an experienced bodybuilder is usually well aware of it when he has not recovered from the previous workout. He feels it. Get acquainted with how you feel the day after a workout. Make notes in your diary or your training log.

The ultimate test of whether a bodybuilder is overtraining is that his progress has come to a halt. But before he concludes that the problem is one of overtraining, he'd better be sure that he is working out on a progressive basis. If not, his no-gain status may be due to laziness or insufficient work.

Schedules

Recuperation from heavy workouts takes up to 48 hours, and therefore daily training for added muscle size is rarely advisable. What is becoming more and more popular among aspiring bodybuilders is the every-other-day split routine. Mentzer follows it, as do numerous other stars. Frank Calta, the noted Florida expert, has a slightly different version, which he calls "rotation for recuperation." He trains half the body every other day, resting Saturdays and Sundays.

Mike Mentzer's every-other-day split works like this: He divides his routine into two and trains half his body on Monday, the other half on Wednesday, the first half again on Friday, and the second half again on Sunday. The next week his workouts would start on a Tuesday. Of course this system is only practical for those who have training facilities available at all times. This system has no respect for the seven-day schedule, known as a week, that man has concocted to pace his style of living.

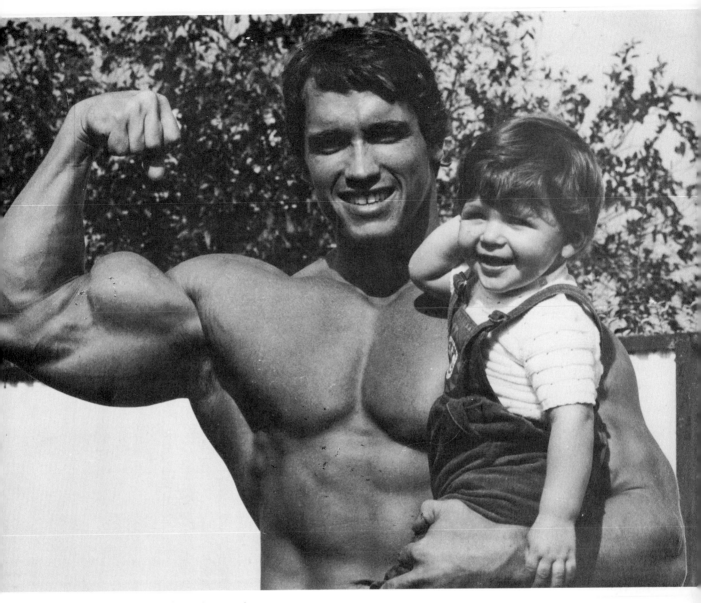

Arnold hams it up with a future champ.

Relaxation

What speeds recuperation? The first answer that comes to mind is relaxation. If one doesn't relax, full recuperation will be greatly prolonged. Many top bodybuilders have learned the art of relaxation. They do it by turning their mind to other interests and enjoyments: art, music, conversation, yoga, poetry, religion, books, or TV.

Most of us respond best to music. Maybe you do, too. So relax, put your feet up, absorb. Spend half an hour with some pretty heavy stuff.

Inspiring and profound music will do a better job at relaxing you than fast beat disco, but the whole point of this soul-washing business is that the music should get its message to *you*, and if "Moonlight Serenade" does things to you, then by all means relax with that. In general, don't be afraid of experiencing deep emotion. You want to be a *whole man*, not merely a muscle machine.

If the Mona Lisa rests your weary mind, get yourself a print. Maybe you like Picasso, Dali, or Van Gogh. Sculptures—Why not? Maybe

Rodin's "The Kiss" or Henry Moore's "Reclining Woman"? Reproductions are available. Then there is Nature's sculpture: fields, streams, mountains, and valleys. What could be more restful?

Do you like poetry? You can read it or listen to it on records as many bodybuilders do. Read some good authors: Thoreau, Wilde, Shaw, Russell, Emerson, Hazlitt, Nietzsche, Goethe. Read about things other than muscles, and your relaxation will pay you dividends.

Some people believe in never running when they can walk, never standing when they can sit, and never sitting when they can lie down. Within limits the hard-working bodybuilder can follow this philosophy. In other words, rest when you can.

Stress

Stress is the enemy of relaxation. Our response to stress is a built-in survival mechanism. When there is a threat to our existence and well-being, our digestive system shuts down, our heart speeds up, breathing deepens, adrenaline and other hormones flood the body to prepare us for fight or flight.

Bertil Fox of Britain always looks for maximum recuperation.

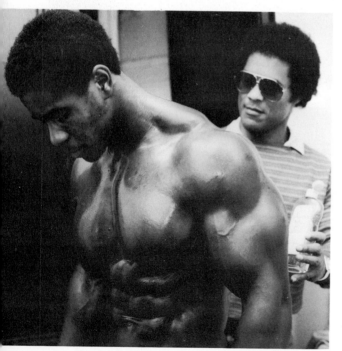

Unnecessary stress leads to wasted energy, and too much of it will stop you from becoming Mr. Olympia. You cannot expect to make regular gains in muscle size if you overwork, overplay, engage in frequent arguments, or burn the candle at both ends. Under that kind of stress, the body does not react to regular training as we would wish. Chronically recurring stress drains the body of energy. The trainer loses his mental concentration and the ability to recover quickly from his workouts.

Sleep

One definite requirement for full recuperation is sleep. As a hard-training, aspiring bodybuilder, you need eight hours of sleep each night. It is possible to get by on less, but it is not ideal. Many bodybuilders keep pretty good hours on weekdays, only to party like crazy over the weekend. Scientists have concluded that we can get too little sleep one night and make up the balance the following night; in other words, we can borrow and pay back sleep, and suffer no adverse consequences. However, such practices are not advisable. Sure you can party once in a while, but make it the exception rather than the rule. For the most part, get those eight hours of sleep every night.

If you have difficulty sleeping because you are overtrained or anxious about an approaching contest, then take a mild sleeping pill, but don't get into the habit of it. Frank Zane has stated that when he can't sleep he takes tryptophane, an amino acid, to help him relax and fall asleep.

Sun and Air

Fresh air and sunshine, often available at the same time, speed up recuperation. I am convinced that this is the one reason why Californian and Floridian bodybuilders make such good progress. Sunshine in moderate doses also stimulates hormone production—a definite plus for the enthusiastic bodybuilder.

Fresh air, deeply breathed, energizes the entire physique. In fact, many consider an athlete's success totally dependent on the amount of oxygen he can ingest. Didn't Arnold Schwarzenegger and Franco Columbu make the best gains of their lives when training at the original

Gold's Gym in Venice Beach, while inhaling pure oxygen from divers' oxygen tanks between heavy sets of grueling barbell exercise? You may personally want to ignore the possibility of fresh air helping recovery, but it is a fact of life. What's certain is that stuffy, centrally heated surroundings are less than ideal for revitalizing the body.

Steroids

Sometimes I hear about the exhausting workout performed by some top-name bodybuilder and I recoil in disbelief. When I actually witness him training though, I have to believe what's going on there, right before my eyes. It should be said here and now that many competitive bodybuilders—weightlifters, strength athletes, and powerlifters, too—can train in this manner because they aid their recuperation by taking artificial steroids. This practice is definitely not recommended. Many serious bodybuilders have become very sick as the result of taking steroids without a proper doctor's prescription and the attendant monitoring of their vital functions.

Being a hard gainer myself, I have been sorely tempted, but have never taken an artificial steroid, not one. Of course, I do have an insight into that subject that few in the sport can equal. As publisher of *MuscleMag International*, I am the steady recipient of mail from readers who have had terrible experiences with these muscle growth drugs. Here's one sample from bodybuilder Hank Zarco:

"I've been a bodybuilder for 31 years. In that time I have experienced all kinds of mishaps from not warming up, overtraining, improper eating, liquor, not enough sleep, and a lack of bodybuilding knowledge. But I still made great gains in strength and muscle quality.

"I was very proud of my strength. Weighing between 142 and 150, I could do 545 pounds in the parallel squat, 2 sets 15 reps; wide chins, 8 sets 8 reps, with 100 pounds around the waist; bent-over row, 3 sets 5 reps, 300 pounds; strict barbell curl, 160 pounds; one-arm French presses, 8 sets 8 reps, 75 pounds.

"But I couldn't stand prosperity. I heard about steroids, and from that point on my health (internal organs) took a downward turn. I wasn't satisfied with the one-a-day prescription. When I gained a few pounds I thought if one

dianabol (5 mg) tablet could do that so soon, what would happen if I increased the dosage?

"For three years I took three 5mg tablets a day. Of course I won Mr. Illinois 1965, Mr. Central USA 1966, Mr. Mid-West 1966, and 2nd Mr. America in the short class (I.F.B.B.), Mr. Colorado 1967, and a total of 67 trophies. But the price was high, because the steroid was beginning to take its effect.

"Every once in a while when I took a few weeks off from the drug, I shrank in muscle size till I went back on it again. Each time it was harder to get back into shape.

"Then my prostate began to suffer till I bled

In the best shape of his life—Lou Ferrigno, the scintillating Hercules.

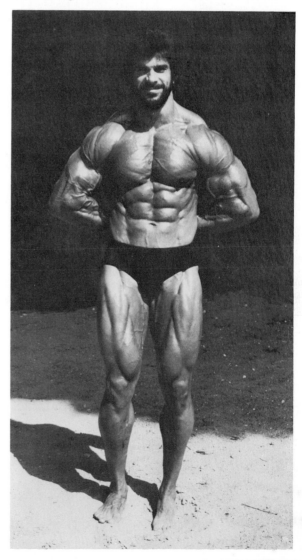

from the penis. Next it was my liver, my kidneys, and my bladder.

"I was forced to stop steroids in 1970. Getting into shape was a chore. I could not get my muscles to respond. Heavy weights hurt me. It took longer to recover, and it seemed as though my tissues were not responding.

"My strength began to lessen each month, until I was using the poundages of a beginner. But I did not give up. I learned humility. I

Scott Wilson—going places in the 80's!

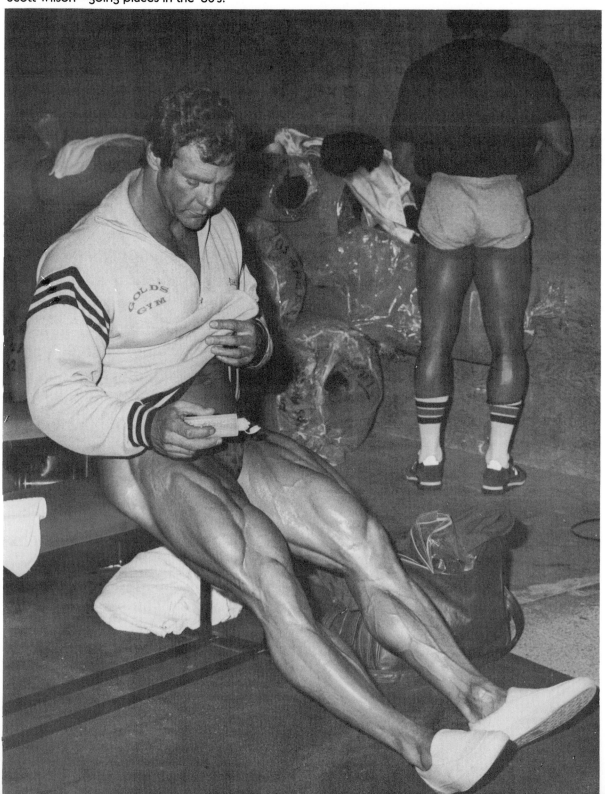

started using better form, more concentration, and the desire to find a better way for better results. This is when better things began to happen to me."

"I found a way for improving a set, exercise, and my own ratio for better recuperation. In short, I developed my own bodybuilding principles. I wish I would have known then what I know today, but that's life. Maybe other bodybuilders can learn from my experience (mistakes). I sure hope so."

Other Drugs and Diversions

There has been some talk recently of the usefulness of Bio-Strath, a yeast-and-herb liquid concentrate imported from Switzerland. According to Caroline Cropp, Nutritional Consultant to Nutrition Vitamin Supplements (Scottsdale, Arizona), exclusive supplier of Bio-Strath in the USA, there are European studies demonstrating that Bio-Strath can increase the amount of oxygen the blood can carry, can give the bodybuilder an increased ability to work hard at the gym, build muscle tone, and improve recovery time.

One controlled test, conducted in Germany, involved test subjects pedaling on stationary bicycles until their heartbeats reached an aerobic level. At that point, measurements were taken to see how long it took for the heart rate to return to normal. The results, according to Cropp: "Significant improvement in recovery time was found in people who were taking Bio-Strath."

Another study showed that rats given Bio-Strath were able to gain more weight on fewer calories. The evidence points to an anabolic (or bodybuilding) effect.

One of our earliest Mr. America's, John Grimek, used to equate bodybuilding with a battleship. If it had a leak, or two or three, then it would sink. "You must seal your leaks," said Grimek, and of course he was right.

The regular use of tobacco and alcohol can be regarded as serious leaks. Both will ultimately affect your physical ability, your mental resolve, and powers of recuperation.

During my many years in bodybuilding, I have known some champions and near champions who were smokers and drinkers. In their first year or two of training, their bad habits didn't appear to be detrimental to their progress.

But then, lo and behold, telltale signs began to show up. I would notice a gradual reluctance to perform heavy, high rep squats and other demanding exercises. That was due to the fact that both cigarettes and booze have a toxic effect, which had worsened and caused nausea during the more vigorous movements. As time went on, their workouts became shorter and their recuperation took longer. Ultimately they could handle no more than an occasional workout, and sometimes only a few exercises. All because booze and nicotine had clogged up the system, tired them out, and robbed them of their vitality.

The so-called recreational drugs are equally harmful, of course. Youngsters can handle things for a while, but the ultimate burn-out is as inevitable as death and taxes. At best, the natural athlete has an up-down career, which eventually nosedives faster than a toboggan. The hard gainer never gets a look in at all.

Many young bodybuilders are concerned about the negative aspects of masturbation. In the not too distant past this was thought to cause everything from madness to blindness. Neither was true, of course, but excessive masturbation can overtire you and may have an adverse effect on your training vitality and general recuperative ability.

Nutrition

The part nutrition can play in maximizing your chance for complete recovery is not to be overlooked. As a rock-bottom minimum, you should have the recommended daily allowance (RDA) of protein, vitamins, and minerals. If you feel that your post-workout recovery proceeds at snail's pace, then I suggest you take a multivitamin (one-a-day type) tablet as general insurance. In addition, you might also benefit from daily doses of a high-quality protein powder mix, B-Complex, vitamins C and E, and some type of chelated mineral supplement.

Bear in mind, too, that if you are trying to gain muscle while losing fat, you may have cut your carbohydrate intake too low. The days of pre-contest starvation are over.

At the very least, your diet should be 100 percent adequate for complete and speedy recuperation. Your recuperation from demanding workouts is of definite importance to your ultimate success. Neglect nothing that can help.

11
BODY FAT PERCENTAGE
The Lean Advantage

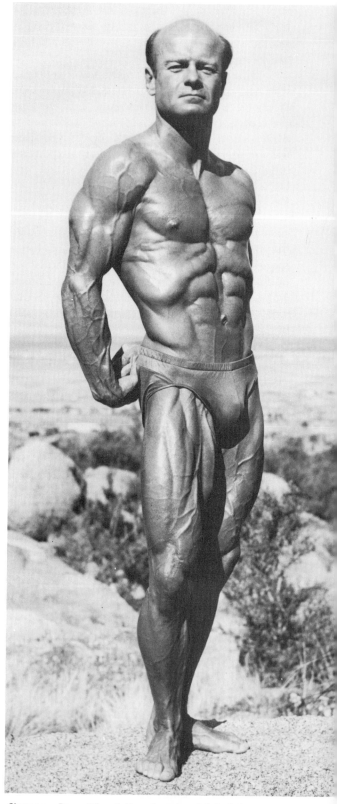

Clarence Bass. His all-time low bodyfat: 2.4 percent!

They used to call it *definition*. Today we use a different term: *bodyfat percentage*.

There is an undeniable movement towards ultimate definition these days, at least around show time. After a contest, things change. Most bodybuilders gain 10 pounds after a contest. Others gain 20, 30, or even 40. Usually, this does not manifest itself as rolls of fat, but as increased overall size and so-called thicker skin. It would be fair to say that you do yourself no good by gaining more than 10 pounds after a show, and if you start to get rolls of fat, you will be in trouble.

When you reduce your fat percentage to less than 7 percent, your body takes on a whole new appearance. Not only do veins show up in minute detail, but cross-striations of the muscles become apparent, so you'll look like an anatomy chart—a picture of muscles with the skin stripped away. That's a condition which has led to a good deal of controversy.

The late David P. Willoughby made constant references to the unsightly appearance of bodybuilders who had an extremely low bodyfat percentage. Nonetheless, most current followers of the sport actually prefer this "ripped" look, and at present writing, it is the fellows with the least fat who are walking away with the top titles in bodybuilding.

The book *Physical Fitness of Champion Athletes*, by Thomas K. Cureton, Jr., computes the average fat percentages of various groups of athletes. Sixteen track and field athletes were found to have 11.88 percent of bodyfat. For fifteen Danish gymnasts, the body average was 10.36 percent, and for twenty-one Olympic swimmers, the average was 10.60 percent. All the groups tested had a median height of 69 inches (1.725 meters) at a weight of 160 pounds, and their average bodyfat content was just under 11 percent.

David Willoughby, who rightly fancied himself as a statistician, came up with a complicated formula in support of his view that very low bodyfat is "downright repellent and creates a disfiguring appearance, which in its extreme emaciation is as unsightly as extreme corpulence." The average man, according to Willoughby, has a bodyfat percentage of 12.56.

John Grimek at 195 pounds bodyweight has a bodyfat ratio of 10 percent. Eugen Sandow has 11.26 percent. Among Olympic and power lifters the percentages are somewhat higher. Doug Hepburn was recorded at 14.07, and Soviet man mountain Vasili Alexeev at 23.70.

With today's champions, unlike those of yesteryear, the bodyfat percentage often fluctuates according to the stage of their training. It is not uncommon for a competitive bodybuilder to cut his bodyfat by two thirds before a contest.

Years ago, an athlete or bodybuilder was praised and honored for possessing a body of harmonious, smooth muscular development. Today the word *smooth* is used solely to deride a bodybuilder for being totally out of shape. Times change.

Incidentally, some of the ancient Grecian statues that presumably represented the Greek ideal of male perfection have also been scrutinized with regard to their bodyfat. The famous Farnese Hercules is estimated to have 11.96 percent, the Apollo Belvedere, 11.76, and Myron's Discobolus 12.06. If these statues were real men, they would probably not do well in the Olympic contest, where the top six men have averaged a bodyfat count of under 5 percent.

Willoughby's thoughts on bodyfat are that the minimum should be 10 percent for men, 20 percent for women, and that ultimate muscularity is ultimate disfigurement. A bodybuilder turned weightlifter who does not share Willoughby's views is Clarence Bass who has to date written two excellent books: *Ripped* and *Ripped 2*. Both report in detail how he achieved ultimate muscularity without undue hunger or pain. Clarence, who got his bodyfat down to 2.4 percent, and even between contests holds his bodyfat down to under 6 percent, rarely indulges in pizza, ice cream, and other high-calorie junk foods. But he does eat cereals, raisins, eggs, and potatoes. Like Zane before him, and Gironda before Zane, Bass has set a trend. Each of these men gave us a new plateau of super-defined appearance.

Tom Platz. His severe training methods pay off.

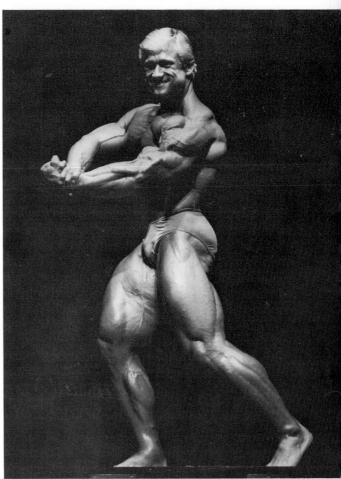

Why does current fashion seem to be pushing the bodybuilding ideal towards being almost fat-free? One reason is that it enables us to see muscles that we never knew we had. Few physique champions of the distant past could show shapely, delineated serratus muscles and incredibly separated thigh muscles. Today you can't even win Mr. America unless all your muscles are diamond sharp. That includes the muscles of the upper thigh and lower back, two areas from which it is difficult to eliminate all fat. Today, fat-free bodies are a must. Maybe styles will once again return to the 11 percent ideal. Who knows. For the moment, however, low fat and cross-striations are the order of the day.

Diet

How do bodybuilders bring their fat down to a very low percentage? One could give an oversimplified answer: they eat less. True enough, but it goes deeper than that!

Most successful body men eat fairly normally when they are not preparing for a contest. That is not to say they eat junk foods. A few do. Most of them don't. As mentioned in another chapter, it is advisable for the food you eat to be as near to its natural state as possible. Foods with natural fibre keep you leaner and fitter than dense calorie foods. Have whole-grain bread, cereals, fruit, vegetables, fish, cheese, organic and white meats, and milk. Stay away from the processed, chemically treated, artificially flavored, brilliantly colored garbage that your local supermarket offers as food.

The theory of losing bodyfat is simple, but it is often difficult for a bodybuilder to follow it in practice. He must progressively cut calories.

Thyroid

Many physique men who do not like to diet rigidly resort to taking a substance named thyroid, which has the effect of speeding up the metabolism. As you may expect, the body's own production of thyroxin will often stop when large doses of thyroid are supplied artificially, even under medical supervision. In many cases, this becomes irreversible, so that the bodybuilder has to take thyroxin artificially for the rest of his life.

Drugs

Another practice is the taking of diuretics in large amounts, mainly a product named LaSix, which makes the body lose large amounts of fluids in a short time. With this fluid, some vital minerals may also be flushed out of the system, for instance potassium, which is needed to regulate the heart beat, among other things. More than one bodybuilder's death has been attributed to the indiscriminate use of diuretics. One star bodybuilder told me in private (accordingly, I will not divulge his name) that he took several tablets of LaSix on the days before a Mr. Olympia event. Then he went on to relate how his body started to burn up on stage. He got cramps in his legs, and it seemed as though he was in a room without air. Ultimately, he gulped water backstage to stop himself from passing out, and for a while he felt that his life was in the balance. Perhaps it was!

Thyomucase is another potentially dangerous drug that bodybuilders have experimented with, all for the vain glory of taking home a $50 trophy! This drug comes in rub-on creams and injectibles. One competitive bodybuilder I know rubbed the cream into his thighs the day before an important show. The result was an unsightly redness and an accompanying painful and severe burn. The fat under his skin, which was supposed to "burn off," stayed.

Vitamins

Choline and inositol, members of the B family of vitamins, are known as aids in the redistribution of fat. At least they are safe and have no known toxic effects—unlike the products I mentioned before.

Choline and inositol can be bought, separately or together, from your local health food store. They were first publicized around 1960, when it was reported that most of the muscle beach stars took these vitamins prior to a contest or posing exhibition. Further experimentation led to the conclusion that choline and inositol appeared to work for the physique contestant if their intake was combined with a strict diet. Certainly, no one could eat like a pig and keep his weight under control simply by taking these substances. However, bodybuilders have lately been adding a new dimension to their training in order to keep their bodyfat down.

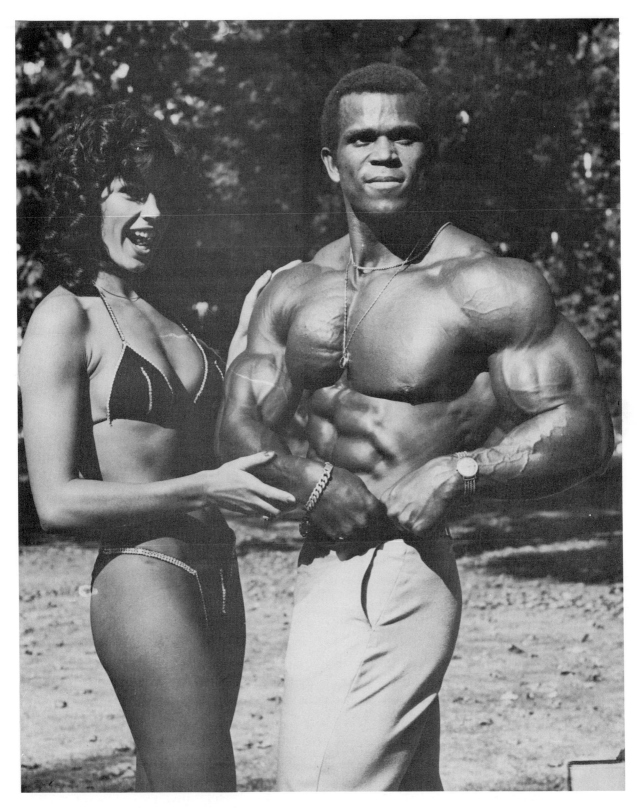

Weight-trained beauty Linda Cheeseman poses with
Serge Nubret, one of the first Europeans to fully utilize
scientific supplementation to greatly reduce bodyfat percent.

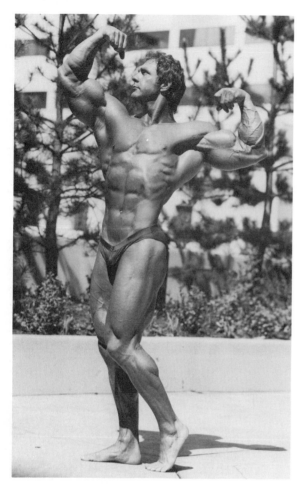

His bodyfat is minimal—Scott Wilson, USA.

Aerobic exercise stimulates the production of enzymes that convert fat to energy. The more fat-burning enzymes you have, the better you can use up or burn excess flab. Not only does aerobic activity burn calories better than anything else, it also increases the body's capacity for burning fat. A long-distance or marathon runner is a veritable fat-burning machine. The reason this is so is that the aerobic activity keeps the heart-pulse rate below 80 percent of your maximum. To estimate your maximum heart rate, subtract your age from 220.

Unlike weight training, which can temporarily boost your heart rate to near maximum, walking keeps your heart rate well under 80 percent of your maximum. According to Bass in *Ripped 2*, walking comes as close as anything to being a pure fat-burning activity.

Needless to say, aerobic exercise should be limited if you are urgently trying to gain weight, and even during regular maintenance training you should not overdo this form of exercise, since it can detract from your bodybuilding gains. Some degree of common sense has to be used so as to balance muscular development with aerobic fitness. If you are fit and well-muscled, you really have a double advantage: extra fat-burning enzymes to help you stay lean, and extra muscle mass.

Gerard Buinoud of France.

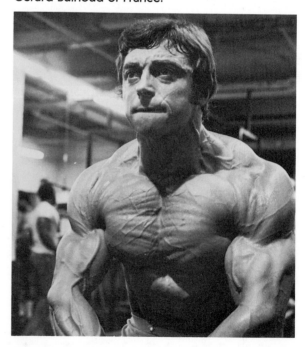

Aerobic Exercise

Weight training may be unparalleled in its potential for building up the skeletal muscles of the body, but is not a particularly good fat-burning activity. Here again, I want to quote Clarence Bass, who has probably more than any one else in competitive bodybuilding made a science of staying lean while holding muscle size. "Aerobic exercise should be included in the program of any bodybuilder interested in staying lean," says Bass. Typical exercise such as stationary bike riding, road cycling, slow jogging, swimming, and walking, burns calories through prolonged, low-intensity effort. Weight training is not aerobic but anaerobic exercise—high-intensity effort which does not result in a steady need for oxygen and a considerably stepped-up heart rate.

Arnold Schwarzenegger at the 1974 Mr. Olympia with Lou Ferrigno.

12
TRAINING THE METABOLISM
Creating the Anabolic State

What is the metabolism? What is your metabolic rate? Is it important to the bodybuilder?

Your metabolism consists of all the chemical processes by which your body produces energy and assimilates new material to maintain, replace, and build up its cells.

Your metabolic rate is the speed at which your body burns up fuel. Your body too has a tick-over speed, just like a car. When it is running fast, it will burn up a great deal of fuel. At a more moderate pace, it uses less fuel.

People have a great many misconceptions about the metabolism and its relationship to bodybuilding. What is important to understand is that the successful bodybuilder does not try, or should not be trying, to speed up his metabolism to a super-accelerated rate (unless he wants to shed fat very quickly), nor does he try to slow down his metabolism to a subnormal level.

In Nature, we can observe two high-metabolism creatures which, due to their genetic makeup, are always in need of food and spend about 95 percent of their waking hours either eating or looking for food. The shrew is in endless pursuit of food, and when you look at this minute creature, you can see its system pumping away and shaking its tiny body like a battery-driven toy. The tiny hummingbird, one of Nature's marvels whose super-fast wing beats enable it to hover in mid-air while stealing its vital nourishment from various plants, is the other insatiable creature. From a study of such high-metabolism creatures we can conclude that a fast metabolism is of little use to the bodybuilder.

So what about a slow metabolism? What creatures can Nature offer us in that direction? The koala bear, the elephant, the rhino, the sloth. A slow metabolism may be conducive to gaining weight, but definitely does not lead to a rapid increase in muscular tissue, which is the ultimate aim of the keen bodybuilder.

There are two aspects to the metabolic process. There is the *anabolic*, or building-up, process, and the *catabolic*, or breaking-down, process. Both processes are constantly taking place in your body. The most desirable state, and one which you can train for, is a positive ratio in favor of the anabolic (building-up) process. As bodybuilding expert John Everett put it in *Iron Man* magazine, "What is required is a positive metabolic ratio."

The Super-Fast Metabolism

Many youngsters are plagued not only by skinniness but by a super-high metabolism. Whatever they do, they just cannot gain weight. Everything they eat is used up in their system. They find it almost impossible to gain weight. Their engines seem always to be running hot!

I have known hundreds, possibly thousands, of these fellows. Even when they drink huge amounts of milk and eat tons of nutritious food, they manage to burn it up. Their weight just does not increase. Then, one fateful (or glorious) day, their metabolism seems to normalize, and suddenly their bodybuilding efforts and generous food intake begin to show results.

Frank Richards, Britain's Mr. Universe, said: "Most Champions get big by learning to slow down their metabolism." OK, so how do we slow down the metabolism? The answer can be summed up in one word: immobilization. The only other way to achieve a slower metabolic rate is by growing older. Our metabolism slows down as we age. Ironically, as we age, it is not a slowing down of our metabolism that we need, but the opposite. Then the fat starts to settle

around our bones, and we yearn for those earlier days when we had an accelerated metabolism.

In order to slow down your metabolism, you must purposely practice relaxation—*real* relaxation. Never run when you can walk. Never walk when you can sit. Don't sit if you can lie. Relaxation, even for ten minutes, is particularly important after a meal.

Try and check on yourself during the day. Are you as relaxed as you can be while you follow your daily routine? How do you watch TV? Do you lean forward in your chair, or do you sit back comfortably with your feet up on a padded stool? Now do you get the idea? Relax! Rid yourself of tension and stress, mental as well as physical.

The Super-Slow Metabolism

If you feel you have a slow metabolism—if you tend to be slow-moving, overweight, and lethargic—you can take steps to stimulate your metabolic processes so as to normalize it. When that begins to happen, your digestive processes will accelerate, your glands will secrete more, and your hormones will be stirred up.

How can you speed up your metabolism? The answer is: by making room in your schedule for exercises that stimulate the metabolism. For a while you will have to put abdominal training, calf work, and arm exercises aside. The true stimulators of our metabolic functions are the movements which work the bigger muscle groups—in other words: squats.

"With poor metabolism you have poor progress," says Peary Rader, who has been preaching specific metabolism training for forty years. "You need to squat with 20 repetitions, and the last 8 repetitions should be forced reps. Make a point of deep breathing between repetitions. You may want to breathe 5 or 6 times for each of the last few reps."

No Recent Progress?

When a bodybuilder has been unable to make any progress at all—especially in his late beginning or early intermediate stages—his gains accelerate enormously as soon as he is placed on a heavy, high-repetition squat program just two days a week. He does not have to use many other exercises. Numerous successful

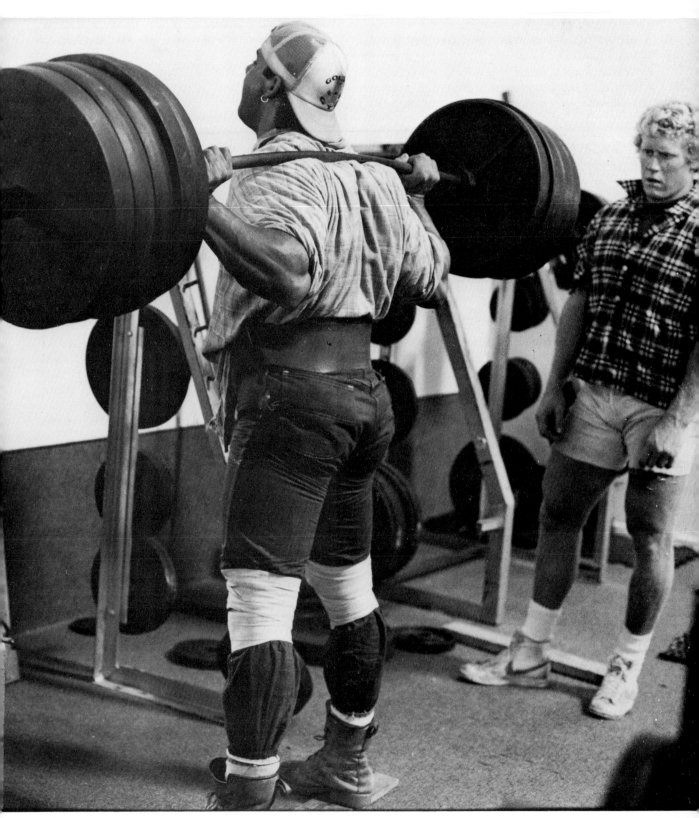

The key metabolism exercise: the squat—
performed Barbarian style.

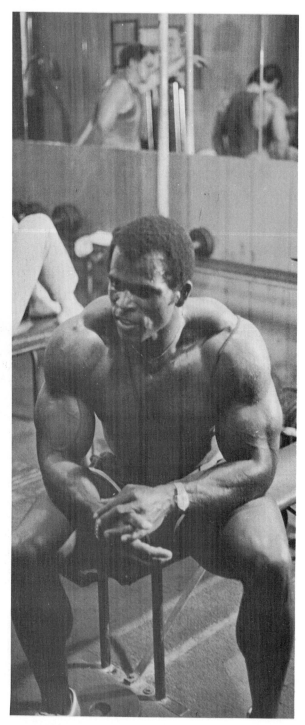

Serge Nubret takes a brief rest.

cases only included the wide-grip chin and bench press along with the squat training for their metabolism.

When an average trainer with a normal metabolism isn't gaining, he will find it helpful

to steer his metabolic ratio towards the anabolic state, for this is needed to build up his body's growth pattern and overall size. That means he should not stay on a heavy, high-rep squatting program for long periods. He should use this form of training to stimulate the metabolism and thereby set the body up for overall gains, but he should alternate it with periods of rest (immobilization) and so allow the body to gain. This is in line with Vince Gironda's system of training (based on thirty years of observing the pupils at his North Hollywood gym), which is to train hard (3–4 times a week) for three weeks, and then to take a complete week's rest.

This, followed by a more normal training routine, will help to favor the anabolic (building-up) metabolism over the catabolic (breaking-down) metabolism.

Virtually all the top bodybuilding champions have used heavy, high-rep squats in their training to give their body overall size. Once this size has been reached, many champs find they don't need those regular, heavy squatting exercises any more. They can get by on hacks, thigh extensions, and other less strenuous leg movements. Ask Frank Zane, Robbie Robinson, Franco Columbu, Samir Bannout. Even when training for a Mr. Olympia title, they may need only four to six weeks of strenuous squatting to bring their thighs and their metabolisms back to peak condition.

Summary

Remember that this metabolism training is not necessary as long as your current bodybuilding routine is developing your muscles at a satisfactory pace. This mode of training is designed specifically for the hard gainer. Virtually all hard gainers who have applied this principle seriously over a period of 3–9 weeks made significant progress, and what is more important, they made this progress when every other form of training had failed.

It should be added here, though I don't want to put a damper on your enthusiasm, that no one can go beyond the limits of his genetic endowment. It is, however, also pretty certain that no Mr. America, Mr. Universe, or Mr. Olympia yet has fully reached the muscle size limits set by his own genetic endowment.

Is it time for you to start squatting?

Favorite bodyman Tom Platz, about to perform a set of lateral raises.

13
ULTIMATE NUTRITION
Musclebuilding and the Food Factor

Until a short while ago, I had never been inside a fast-food restaurant. Can you believe it? Probably not. But it's true. Fast foods were something I avoided. It's not that I am a food fanatic. That I have never been, but I have always tried to eat what is considered *good* food. For the most part, anyway.

Well I've got news for you. Virtually all the fast-food establishments I have seen are peddlers of complete and utter junk. After tasting their wares and being physically sick, I wouldn't even feed my cat that stuff. In fact, my cat couldn't be persuaded to eat it if it were mixed with the finest, flaky white tuna!

Tough talk? You bet! Who wants to fill his stomach with sodium and sugar, high fat, and chemical additives? Anything that is so highly processed does not make good sense nutritionally.

In spite of the fact that one or two top bodybuilders have made it to the Olympia by eating more than their share of junk food, the serious bodybuilder of the competition platform must be disciplined about the foods he eats. Today this is so more than ever before, because it's the low bodyfat, thin skin, and manifest definition that wins today's contests. You will not achieve this condition and couple it with a generous degree of muscle mass without adhering strictly to a proper diet.

Together with progressive resistance exercise and adequate rest, nutrition is a vital requirement for bodybuilding success. There is the accepted notion now that "we are what we eat," so trillions of words have been written about food and diet. The ideas they propound run the entire gamut from the acceptance of junk food to the necessity of almost eternal fasting. Needless to say, neither extreme is recommended.

Your muscles are made up of about 70 percent water and 20 percent protein. However, the practice of greatly increasing your intake of either water or protein, or both, will not increase your muscle size. It will simply cause the body to excrete more water or protein, or both. In other words: enough is enough!

Traditionally, bodybuilders have gone in for eating huge amounts of protein—steaks, cheese, poultry, fish, eggs, nuts, and of course protein supplements. But with the advent of Dr. Nathan J. Smith's tome *Food for Sport*, and his

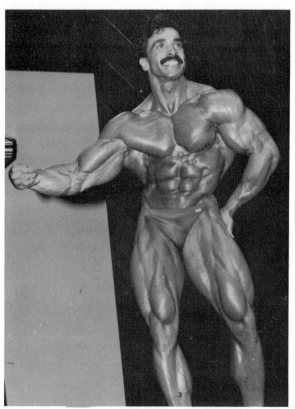

Samir Bannout got ripped by following the principles of good nutrition.

statement, "It is important for athletes to recognize that their athletic activity, although it may require a high energy expenditure, will not significantly increase their need for protein," the protein-overload theory has lost some of its popularity. But let us not overreact. Even the most enthusiastic member of the low-protein brigade has to admit that the would-be champion bodybuilder does indeed need more protein than the layman, or even the competitive athlete. Here's the point, though, and affirmed by no lesser authorities than bodybuilding researchers Clarence Bass and Mike Mentzer: "Only a little more than the usual amount of protein is required for muscle-building purposes."

Protein is the least efficient source of energy, and ironically, too much of it may result in a slower rate of recovery and give you superfluous calories that turn into fat. It is far better to concern yourself with a high-carbohydrate diet.

Yes, carbohydrate is the main fuel for muscles. It becomes glucose in the blood and is stored by your muscles and organs in the form of glycogen. During and after concentrated workouts, your glycogen becomes depleted. Since your recovery is largely dependent on the restoration of glycogen in the muscles, a diet high in carbohydrate speeds the restoration process.

According to Clarence Bass in his excellent book *Ripped*, "studies have shown that a high carbohydrate diet fully restored the glycogen in the muscles after 48 hours, while a high protein and fat diet left glycogen levels below par even after five full days. Clearly, a diet high in carbohydrate does the job of getting you ready for your next workout."

Vince Gironda is always talking about "positive nitrogen balance," another term for taking in more protein than we lose. This is a definite "must" for the aspiring bodybuilder, because a negative nitrogen balance would have us losing muscle size.

How much protein do we need to grow? Actually, musclebuilding is a relatively slow process, so we don't need all that much. For a 154-pound man, the National Research Council sets its recommended daily allowance of protein at 70 grams (1 gram per 2.2 pounds of bodyweight). That is a very generous allowance, since some studies have shown that people can keep very healthy on a considerably smaller intake of protein. In other words, it is unlikely that

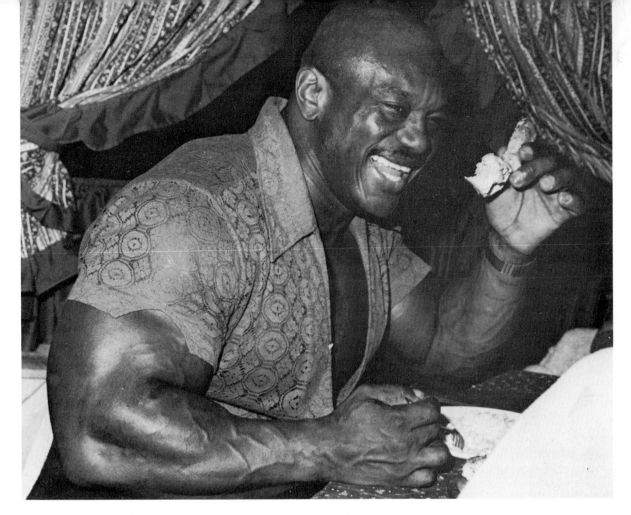

The incredible Sergio Oliva. Eating is one of his great loves.

a bodybuilder will need more than 1 gram of protein for each 2.2 pounds of bodyweight. But if you take more, then do it sparingly. This will not only help to keep the fat off, but it will also save you a bundle of money.

Lest you think I have a particular "down" on protein, let me be the first to state that you don't need a great deal of *any* extra food—protein, fat, or carbohydrate—when you are trying to gain muscle. What is important, is that you eat frequently. Five or six small meals are infinitely superior to three large gut-bustin' gourmet extravaganzas. Small meals maintain your blood sugar level on an even keel, keep you from getting hungry, and prevent the discomfort of digesting large, ungainly meals. It is an antiquated concept to stuff oneself with food to gain weight. The result will invariably be added fat, not muscle.

Of course there are people who must eat a lot. For example, if a budding weight trainer has

a high metabolism (the rate at which his body burns fuel while resting), his food intake must be tailored accordingly. If you burn up 3,000 calories in a day, then something more than those 3,000 will be needed for you to gain weight. There are individuals who require 5,000 calories a day. If they eat more than that, they will gain weight. If they eat less than that, they will lose weight. The art is to find out by trial and error how many calories you need to gain or lose weight slowly. Doing either too quickly will give less satisfactory results.

It is generally accepted that a person who leads a moderately active life has a daily need of about 15 calories per pound of bodyweight. Your food intake should maximize your chances of bodybuilding success. Misuse your nutritional regimen, and you will either fail to gain muscle mass, or else you will cover what muscle mass you do develop with an unattractive layer of fat!

A balanced diet (how many times have you

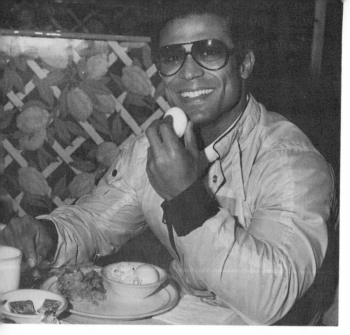
Handsome Mohamed Makkawy partakes of a couple of boiled eggs and a green salad, his pre-contest diet.

heard this phrase?) is the best way to gain lean muscle mass, muscle without the encumbrance of fat. It is true that a balanced diet can mean different things to different people, but in essence it should include nutrition from each of the following food groups:

1. Milk (milk, yogurt, cottage cheese, cheese, etc.)
2. Meat (beef, veal, lamb, pork, fish, poultry, eggs, etc.)
3. Vegetables (fruits, vegetables, legumes, nuts)
4. Grains (bread, cereals)
5. Fats (butter, margarine, oils)

About 65 percent of your diet should be made up of grains, fruits, and vegetables; the remaining 35 percent should come from the milk and meat groups.

So far we have two things to consider: (a) We must balance our diets by eating foods from all five groups every day. (b) We must consume the right number of calories to effect either a weight gain or a weight loss (unless, of course, we simply want to maintain the status quo).

Calories are important, of course, but do not simply choose a program of low-calorie foods when you want to lose weight, or of high-calorie foods when you want to gain weight. *Foods should never be evaluated solely by their calories.* Dr. Jean Mayer of the Harvard School of Nutrition says: "A proper diet must provide all necessary nutrients in sufficient amounts, be palatable, easily available from the viewpoints of economics and convenience, and be balanced in calories to produce the desired caloric deficit for weight loss or additional storage for weight gain."

You must aim for the best possible return for every calorie consumed, and that is why you must avoid "calorie-dense foods" for the greater part of your life. Calorie-dense foods are those unforgivable concoctions prepared or manufactured to appease the whims of taste, with little or no regard for balanced nutrition or sensible nourishment. Calorie-dense foods richly deserve the title *junk food*, and are characterized by their obscene preponderance of chemical additives, coloring, and preservatives—not to mention their lunatic levels of those two demons, salt and sugar.

As the name suggests, calorie-dense foods provide calories in abundance, but they do not really satisfy the appetite. As a result, you tend to overeat, for the more you eat of this garbage, the more you want!

Sugar and butter are perfect examples of calorie-dense foods, and one way or another, they appear in abnormal quantities in just about every food man has attempted to "improve." Other calorie-dense foods (though to my mind they hardly merit the name *food*) are gravies, cream, jam, canned fruit, pastry, cookies, shortening, candy, chocolate, jelly, soft drinks, vegetable oil, processed cheese, potato chips, regular breakfast cereals, salad dressing, canned soup, ketchup, ice cream, crackers, and virtually all prepackaged variety store specials.

It's always amazing to me how a natural, wholesome product such as bread can be devitalized by reducing its natural vitamin content, removing its bulk fibre, bleaching it, dosing it with preservatives so it stays squeezy-fresh on the shelf, and adding Vitamin D or whatever, and is then claimed to be "vitamin-enriched."

Most foods, especially processed foods, seem designed not to maximize health or satisfy your hunger and nutritional needs, but to create a craving for more of the same. Why else would the manufacturers pander to the "sweet-tooth" weakness of the human race by adding sugars and artificial flavorings in such sickening abundance?

Most packaged or canned foods are processed and to be classed as calorie-dense. They stimulate, rather than satisfy, your appetite. They move through your system poorly, are totally unbalanced nutritionally, and make you want to overeat (and get fatter by the day). How government can allow the big food companies of the world to continue screwing up Nature's formulas (and our systems) is beyond me. Until the authorities have the sense to legislate this nutritional hocus-pocus out of our lives, you'll have to watch out for yourself and keep away from all calorie-dense junk foods.

Realizing that all food, if eaten in sufficient quantity, could make one fat, man has sought to invent a satisfying calorie-free food. Little did he realize that Nature in her wisdom had beaten him to it millions of years ago. High-fibre foods are almost always low in calories, because fibre contains almost no calories! Yes, that's right. Fibre is almost calorie-free. There's more.

A high-fibre food requires more chewing; it's not digested, yet helps to satisfy your hunger as it reaches the large intestine, where only a minimal amount of calories are absorbed through the intestinal wall. High-fibre foods are the "miracle foods" that man couldn't invent. They control calorie consumption and actually reduce the number of calories you absorb from the other foods that you eat. The more you keep to high-fibre nutrition, the leaner you're likely to be, and with a lower percentage of body fat, your muscle mass will be more impressive.

Now that you understand the value of fibre and the worthlessness of calorie-dense junk foods (which are loaded with fat, sugar, and zillions of unpronounceable additives), change your nutritional habits around and try to eat correctly. The best sources of dietary fibre are whole grains, fruits, and vegetables. Does that sound paradoxical? Did you expect me to give you a list of magical new names? There aren't any. What you must realize is that when I say *whole grains*, I mean whole grains. A cereal label may claim that a product is made from pure, wholesome wheat or corn, but this does not mean that it is unadulterated. More than 90 percent of the packaged breakfast cereals are simply overpriced, sugar-loaded junk. Read the labels.

In the same vein, do not think that canned fruits are acceptable to our cause. They are not. Look at the sugar content. What about those other additives?

Do not drink fruit juices if you want to keep your bodyfat content low. They pass straight into the bloodstream and are very easily stored as fat—and where's the fibre? Did you throw it away when you squeezed out your nectar? Probably. Far better to eat an apple in the way nature intended, with all its fibre, than to down a glass of crystal-clear, store-bought apple juice. Where's the fibre?

Bread and potatoes are invariably singled out as fattening foods; and served the way most people eat them, they are! Most bread is devitalized and not worth the pan it's been baked in. Apart from that, we have the habit of covering it with calorie-dense butter and sugar-loaded jams, jellies, or marmalades. But by itself, whole-wheat bread made with natural ingredients is a particularly useful food to the bodybuilder and should be eaten in moderation every day. However, even whole-wheat breads may have added sugar and salt, so look at the labels to avoid these ingredients.

It's the same thing with potatoes. We submerge them in fat and make them into french fries, or serve them with butter or sour cream. A baked potato, as opposed to the greasy french fry, is nutritionally sound. But please hold the butter and sour cream if you want to have a low fat percentage. Your fat intake—and make no mistake about it, some fat is needed in the diet—can come from other sources, such as milk.

Champion bodybuilder Ali Mala tempts Canada's Reid Schindle to a plate of tasty healthfood.

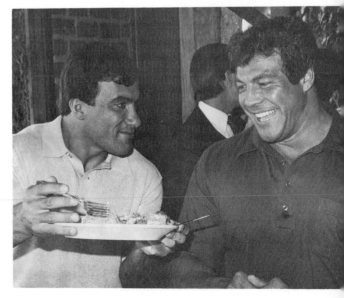

Yes, milk. You should drink some of it every day. That is not to say you should drink gallons of it, but milk is a wonderful nutrient. Some people cannot digest it because of lactose intolerance. They can add the enzyme lactose to their milk. A product called Lact-Aid is made for this purpose and can be bought at drug stores, pharmacies, and health food stores.

Not just babies, but adults, too, should drink milk because it is high in calcium. To the bodybuilder, this mineral is very important: it keeps your bones strong. It also helps your heart to pump and your brain to think, and is vital for muscle contractability. If your body is not supplied with adequate calcium (3 glasses of milk a day is recommended), it will rob your bones or your teeth for its supply. A regular calcium deficiency can cause osteoporosis (weakening of the bones), a disease suffered by 15 million North Americans.

Foods other than milk that are high in calcium include yogurt, cheddar cheese, green leafy vegetables (collards, broccoli, mustard greens, cabbage, kale, spinach), dried beans, almonds, and brazil nuts.

An enemy of the bodybuilder, especially when he is trying to cut up before a contest, is sodium. Yes, the dreaded salt. In fact, it may be the arch enemy of mankind. Certainly, too much of it predisposes one to high blood pressure. I recall Dr. Albert Schweitzer stating that he felt an excessive salt intake was one of the principal causes of cancer in humans.

The bad news for bodybuilders is that one part of sodium holds 180 parts of water. This may explain how some bodybuilders, in spite of rigorous calorie reduction, can come into a contest looking bloated and, yes, waterlogged! Clearly, a little sodium makes a big difference.

A good rule for the bodybuilder, and for the health enthusiast, is to use table salt very sparingly. All people require salt for normal health, but our daily requirement is extremely low. In fact, deficiencies are rare because most of our foods contain sodium. You will probably get quite enough from ordinary, untreated fruits and vegetables.

It is quite safe to say that many people take in over three hundred times more salt than they need. Why? The answer lies partly in its function as a preservative. Like sugar, salt helps to prevent food from going bad. So sodium is pumped into just about every edible thing available. Check the labels, and there it is: *Sodium*. A McDonald's Big Mac contains 1,510 milligrams of sodium, and a Kentucky Fried Chicken has 2,128 milligrams. When you consider that the average person often adds more salt to these items, and then even more as he douses his fast foods with ketchup or other sodium-loaded sauces, you can assume that millions of people eat between 5,000 and 15,000 milligrams of sodium a day. Even cottage cheese, a long-time "food of the bodybuilder," contains 850 milligrams of sodium in just one cup.

Many bodybuilders have the innate (or should I say inane?) conception that more is *always* better, and they apply this not only to their muscle size but also to their food intake. The problem is, of course, that sooner or later more food leads to more fat. Fat is one of the bugs that no physique man wants to contend with, because he will sooner or later be faced with the arduous task of getting it off! There is absolutely no evidence to support the theory that gaining fat hastens muscle growth. Stuffing yourself with

Rod Koontz concentrates on triceps pressdowns at World's Gym. He believes in ultra-nutrition without the use of artificial steroids.

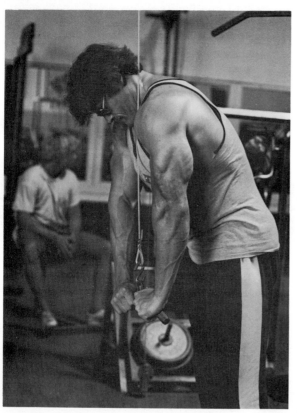

every food in sight will help you to gain weight (a dubious achievement in itself), but there is no advantage whatsoever in providing your muscles with more nourishment than they require at any particular time.

In bodybuilding you must be realistic. A gain of one pound of lean muscle each month is commendable, certainly after the first year of bodybuilding, but is extremely rare. If you train hard enough (and that is the first requirement), then it is possible, by applying a few nutritional facts, to calculate roughly how many calories and grams of protein you will need to achieve a monthly gain of one pound of lean muscle.

Simply put, a pound of muscle contains 600 calories; a pound of fat contains 3,500. There are, as you can see, many more calories in a pound of fat, and fat development requires no outward stimulation, such as the progressive exercise needed to generate muscle. The reason why fat contains so many more calories than muscle is that the water content of fat is only 15 percent, while muscles contain some 70 percent. There is also a wide difference in lipids (cell components high in calories) between the two. Muscle contains only 6 percent lipids. Fat contains 70 percent lipids.

To stimulate one pound of muscle growth each month and make a total gain of twelve pounds in a year, you would have to increase your calorie intake by 600 (the number of calories in a pound of muscle) multiplied by 12 (the number of months in a year), or 7,200 calories a year over and above the amount needed for current weight maintenance. This is 7,200 calories in one year, not one day. To ascertain how many additional calories you require daily to gain pure muscle at this rate, simply divide 7,200 by 365 (the number of days in a year) and you'll come up with approximately 19 extra calories a day. Yes, that's all you need to develop additional lean mass at the rate of one pound a month! It may be worthwhile to exceed this amount for insurance, but not by a large margin. Otherwise you may become fat!

For all the reasons I have just given, I do not agree with the concept of bulking up. By definition, bulking means the addition of size and weight at any cost, even though most of it will be fat. This was done in the old days of bodybuilding. When I first became interested in bodybuilding, my introduction to the nutritional side of the sport came from a Charles Atlas

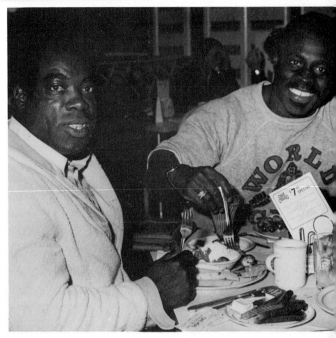

Watch out, Johnny Fuller—Roy Callendar is swiping your grub!

course. I was a mere kid then, living in Britain. The course recommended that one drink several quarts of milk each day, plus a generous supply of eggs, fresh citrus fruits, and daily steaks. At the time, this advice could have come from Mars or Jupiter. Post-war rationing was still in effect, and most Britishers were limited to six ounces of meat per week! Eggs were a rarity, and I for one, had never seen a grapefruit, an orange, or a lemon!

When rationing was removed, every bodybuilder in Britain went crazy. Milk was the main bulking secret. It was the "steroid" of that era— the secret of success. Many a bodybuilder put on twenty or thirty pounds drinking milk. It was drunk before, during, and after meals, right until bedtime. The gains came like magic. Only later did we realize that more than half of what we'd gained was fat. No matter, we refused to believe it and simply changed the name to *bulk*.

I know that many men prefer the bulked-up look. They do not like definition. They just want to be big. If this is your idea of perfection, then simply drink a quart of milk two hours after each meal. Train two times a week for an hour and a half on six basic exercises: *the press behind neck, squat, barbell rows, bench press, curls, and parallel-bar dips.* Presto, you will get bulk—and you're welcome to it.

Nutrition can be as simple or complicated as you want to make it. Animals seem to have no problem. They don't know a vitamin from a calorie, but their instinct guides them to do the right thing. Many humans ingest all kinds of foods that their cat would refuse without hesitation. Some of the healthiest people around have no knowledge of what constitutes good nutrition. Conversely, many well-informed people make horrendous mistakes.

To recap: When a bodybuilder wants to gain weight, he must make sure he selects foods from the various food categories and eats sufficiently to nourish his muscles. Of course, he must also see to it that his body is subjected to vigorous, *progressive* resistance every 48 hours.

To lose fat, you must continue to exercise so as to maintain the status quo of muscle development while progressively restricting your overall calorie intake. In addition, you have to watch your sodium intake.

Not Recommended!

Here's a typical daily menu of the *average* North American:

Breakfast

	Calories
1 large glass orange juice or corn flakes	120
3 slices bacon	78
2 eggs fried in butter	202
2 slices white bread with butter and jam	275
Meal Total	675

Lunch

Big Mac	561
French fries	214
12 oz. cola	145
Meal Total	920

Dinner

	Calories
4 oz. T-bone steak	535
Baked potato with pat of butter	240
½ cup peas	56
Side salad, 1 tbsp. thick dressing	165
Apple pie and ice cream	395
Meal Total	1,391
Meal Total for the Day	2,986

Snacks, gum, beer, candies, etc., can easily add another 600–800 calories.

Recommended

Now here is a typical natural fibre menu for a day:

Early Morning Snack

	Calories
½ grapefruit	45

Breakfast

1 cup oatmeal or rolled oats	130
1 tbsp. raisins	80
2 tbsp. bran	33
1½ cups raw whole milk	225
1 sliced apple	100
Meal Total	613

Lunch

Two-egg whole-wheat sandwich (no butter)	224
Mixed salad, 1 bowl (squeezed lemon to add taste)	150
1 orange	65
1 cup plain yogurt	150
Meal Total	589

Mid-Afternoon

1 oz. cheddar cheese (1-inch cube)	116
2 oz. unsalted cashews or peanuts	200

Dinner

1 whole breast broiled chicken	310
1 baked potato (no butter or sour cream)	90
1 cup green beans	30
2 whole steamed carrots (medium size)	40
1 cup fruit salad (no sugar, any combination of strawberries, tangerines, peaches, banana, blueberries, raspberries, grapefruit, apples, pineapple)	80
Meal Total	866

Evening Snack

1 bran muffin	85
1½ cups whole milk	225
Meal Total	310
Meal Total for the Day	2,378

Here is another ideal menu for the day:

Early Morning Snack	**Calories**
1 banana	120

Breakfast	
2 boiled eggs	160
2 tbsp. raisins	160
2 slices whole wheat bread	144
1 cup mixed fruit salad	80
1½ cups milk	225
Meal Total	889

Lunch	
3 oz. cold, sliced, lean roast beef	250
1 oz. cheddar cheese (1″ cube)	116
1 medium tomato	35
2 carrot sticks	20
1 celery stick	5
1 slice whole-wheat bread	72
1 large apple	120
2 glasses water	0
Meal Total	618

Mid-Afternoon Snack	
1 carrot-raisin muffin	85
1½ cups milk	225

Dinner	
Fresh vegetable soup (1 bowl)	100
Salmon steak (6 oz)	300
Brown rice (½ cup)	100
Broccoli (2 stalks)	90
Fresh corn	70
2 broiled tomatoes	70
1 cup plain yogurt with tangerine slices	190
Meal Total	1,230

Evening Snack	
1 banana	120
Meal Total for the Day	2,857

A wholesome natural diet is far more filling than the average diet, and infinitely superior nutritionally. Forget processed, chemically treated junk foods. You just don't need added preservatives, coloring, and fresheners, and you can do without fried and canned foods. Keep it natural and fresh! Stay away from calorie-dense foods.

Supplementing Your Diet

What about supplements? Are they needed? This can be a pretty tough question. Most top bodybuilders have supplemented their food intake heavily. Yet, there are some like Mike Mentzer and Arnold Schwarzenegger who only take supplements before an important contest. A few take no supplements whatsoever.

It certainly is a good idea to take a good vitamin/mineral one-a-day pill when you are dieting to lose weight or gain definition. This is one time when your body could otherwise become deficient in some substances. Since one-a-day type vitamins cost only pennies a day, I am in favor of taking them regularly. That will be some kind of insurance against having your training undermined. Soviet athletes invariably have their blood tested for possible vitamin deficiencies while they are training for competition, and they are quite often found to be in need of certain minerals or vitamins. Then supplementation is given right away, and they are back in balance. If you are deficient, your training achievements are adversely affected.

You can actually get too much of some vitamins, specifically A and D; they can make you vomit or give you diarrhea, so do not take them in more than the recommended dose. If you want to take larger doses of vitamins, then you might like to experiment with taking extra Vitamins C, B, and E.

Vitamin C

This water-soluble vitamin is useful in aiding tissue repair (after heavy workouts) and helps to protect against infection (colds and flu) and the pollution most of us are subjected to. It helps to heal wounds, burns, and bleeding gums, promotes healing after surgery, and plays a part in decreasing blood cholesterol.

There is evidence to show that a high, regular intake of Vitamin C acts as a natural laxative, lowers the incidence of blood clots in the veins, and extends life by enabling protein cells to hold together. According to Dr. Linus Pauling, it may also decrease cancers by 75 percent, if taken in daily doses of 1,000 to 10,000 mg.

Most animals can actually produce Vitamin C, but man, apes, and guinea pigs must rely upon dietary sources. It is used up at a faster rate by smokers, older people, and those constantly under stress.

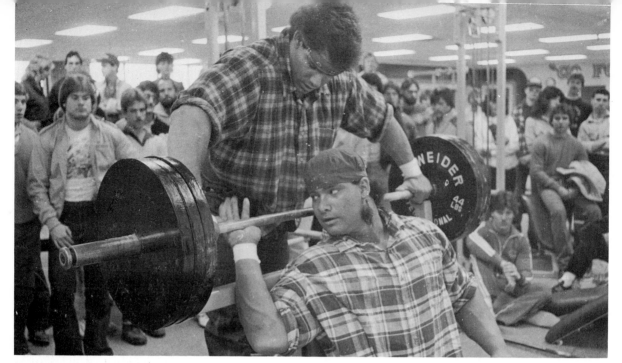
Barbarians Peter and David Paul know the importance of heavy training and ultimate nutrition.

The best natural sources for Vitamin C are citrus fruits, berries, rose hips, green and leafy vegetables, cauliflower, potatoes, and tomatoes.

B Vitamins
Like Vitamin C, all B vitamins are water-soluble, so they should be supplied every day. They also are *synergistic* (more potent together than separately). B_1, B_2, and B_6 should be equally balanced (e.g., 50 mg. B_1, 50 mg. B_2, and 50 mg. B_6) to work effectively.

The Vitamin B family has highly beneficial effects on the nervous system and on mental attitude. It can promote growth, aid digestion, help to keep your heart and skeletal muscles functioning normally, and normalize energy levels. If you drink alcohol regularly, or coffee, you may need Vitamin B-complex supplementation.

The best natural sources of B vitamins are dried yeast, whole wheat, oatmeal, peanuts, bran, most vegetables, milk, and rice husks.

Vitamin E
Vitamin E is stored in the body for only a relatively short time, so it should be supplied every day.

By retarding cellular aging due to oxidation, it may keep your looks younger and may also improve your endurance. Vitamin E can also prevent or dissolve blood clots and lower your blood pressure by working as a diuretic.

The best natural sources for this vitamin include wheat germ, soy beans, broccoli, brussel sprouts, spinach, whole-wheat breads, eggs, whole-grain cereals, and vegetable oils.

Protein Powders
If you want to supplement your protein intake with a protein mix one or two times daily, make sure you choose a high-quality product. It does not matter when you take your protein mix, as long as you realize that the body cannot assimilate more than 25 grams at any one time. Most champions choose a milk-and-egg powder, which they mix in a blender for a few seconds with milk or some other nutritious liquid.

According to Dr. Michael Walczak, who is the nutritional adviser to numerous top California-based bodybuilding stars, a beef-gland (meat) protein could be even better because its amino acids are in the exact proportion you need for your own glands to function correctly. Vince Gironda was one of the first to recommend desiccated beef-liver tablets for ultimate bodybuilding success.

Whether you choose beef-gland or milk-and-egg protein supplementation, remember that you do not need gigantic amounts. You get (or should get) plenty of protein from your regular nutrition, so your protein supplement only acts as a booster to your overall nutrition program. Too much could result in added fat!

14
DERAILING THE STICKING POINT
Regulating the Physiological Processes

Seven-time Olympian Arnold Schwarzenegger. He would train every day for a top contest.

What happens when, after a lay-off, you jump right into hardcore bodybuilding? It happens to every guy without exception! The answer is that you gain muscle size rapidly. But there's more. After growing like crazy for a while, your growth rate will slow down and finally stop altogether. You can continue to go all out, eat well, rest sufficiently, but the answer is always the same: you're stuck! Nothing happens. Your muscles just do not want to grow bigger. This reaction is far from unusual. It is no exaggeration to say that 95 percent of all active bodybuilders are currently at a "sticking point" in their training.

Progressive resistance exercise is a stress, and when you first subject your body to this form of stress it reacts quickly, getting itself ready for further stress by strengthening and enlarging its muscles and tendons. But the body will only do so much. It will not continue to add muscle size unless there is a very good reason. Merely repeating what you first did to stress or shock the body is not enough to keep your body growing

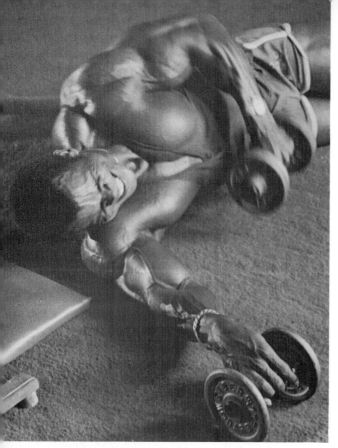

Shock treatment: Nubret performs set after set of lateral raises while lying on the floor.

go will never build super-large muscles. If you are the type who plays tennis before your workout and goes dancing afterwards, then wave goodbye to those 20-inch guns you wanted for Christmas. They won't come this year, or next, or ever!

Of course, this applies also to extra sports activities. By all means bodybuild and engage in sports, but when the time comes that you want to maximize your gains, then your extra activities must go. Later, when you have achieved your goal, you can bring them back into your calendar.

Even today with split and double-split routines, most bodybuilders find it most beneficial to train only every other day, leaving a complete day of rest after each workout.

Barbell and dumbbell training is the most severe form of exercise man has invented to punish his muscles. Bench press 200 pounds 10 times, and in a mere matter of seconds you have lifted some 2,000 pounds! See what I mean? Believe me, after a complete weight training workout in which you will likely lift hundreds of tons via your repeated sets and repetitions, you will need . . . rest.

Shock Treatment

Mohamed Makkawy was having trouble building his back. In the relaxed position it just didn't compare favorably with the likes of Robby Robinson, Tony Pearson, and Greg DeFerro. He didn't know what to do. Heavy rowing hurt his lower back, and he was already doing loads of chins. After talking the problem over with Vince Gironda, the Iron Guru took a couple of days and then mailed Mohamed not *one* back routine but *three!* "To be followed in succession: a different one each back workout," said Vince. "It will keep your muscles guessing."

Reg Park, writing in *MuscleMag International*, said that in order to get his calves to respond, he had to "jolt" them with a different routine every day.

Stubborn muscles must be surprised frequently to budge them out of complacency and to get them to grow bigger and bigger. Arnold Schwarzenegger: "I change around my exercises from time to time, and even perform them in a different manner . . . to shock my muscles into growing."

and growing. New stresses or shocks have to be found.

Before I go any further with this, I should point out that it is entirely unreasonable to expect your muscles to keep growing steadily all the time. There just *have* to be periods of slow or nonexistent growth. At such times, the muscles consolidate their gains; they may even lose a fraction. But you should look upon sticking points with some tolerance. These plateaus are periods in which the body is taking stock and building a base from which you can leap to the *next* level of muscular achievement.

Yes, sticking points are OK, providing (a) they don't happen too frequently, and (b) they don't last too long. However, overly frequent and overly long sticking points can be avoided.

Rest

If you do not allow your muscles sufficient time to recover after a workout, you will dig yourself into an almighty staleness that will be difficult to shake. A person who is always on the

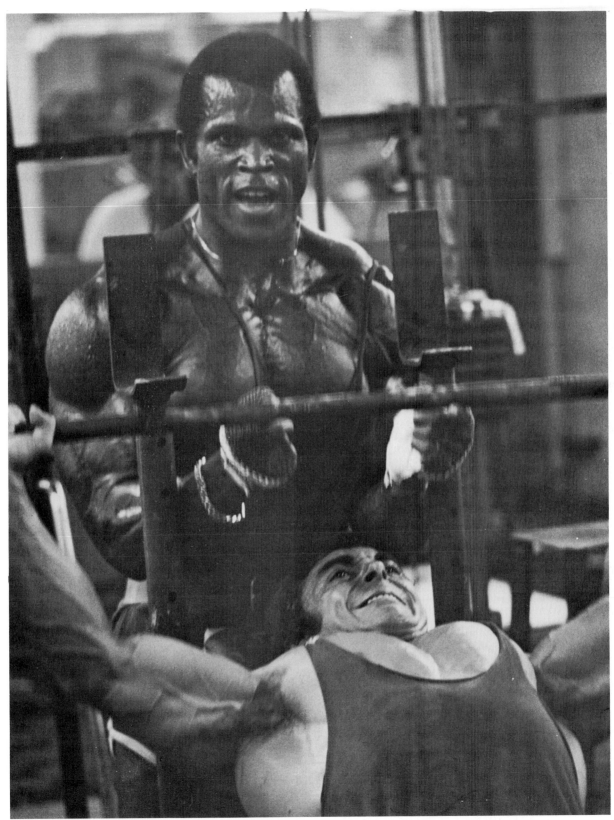

Serge Nubret and his friend Gerard Buinoud help each other's progress by training together.

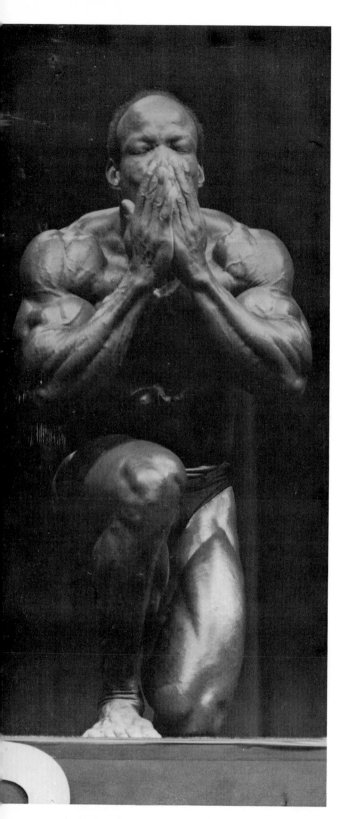

Al Beckles has been getting better every year for over thirty years.

Sameness leads to boredom. Variety will bring about reaction. Of course, one could try to shock the muscles by never performing the same routine twice. Steve Reeves reportedly followed this philosophy to some degree. However, the general consensus is that one's schedule should be repetitive to some extent in order to stimulate regular exercise progression. It is when the fullest intensity has been extracted from a particular exercise that the muscle must be "shocked" into responding. You must, in some deviously planned manner, overwhelm it with a complete change of pace, a new exercise, considerably more or fewer repetitions, a change in your exercise sequence, or in the frequency of your workouts, or some other new mode of training. The prime requisite is that the change be sufficient to make your muscles react.

Lay-offs

Like anything else, lay-offs are good if used properly. If you lay off from training too frequently though, that will most probably doom you to failure, but there are many good reasons why you should lay off from time to time. A few days rest—a week if need be—gives your body time to accumulate nutritional and nervous energy; for here's my point: *The body must be in positive condition to benefit from exercise.*

Your body's reaction to progressive weight training is what it's all about. You may train extremely hard and yet not gain for reasons *other* than exercise. Your reaction to heavy exercise may be nil (and after a couple of months of training, this is what it's most likely to be), because you *never* give yourself a chance to benefit from exercise. Timely lay-offs can keep your muscles growing.

Workout Duration

Gradually increasing the length of your workout (without increasing the length of rests between exercises) can serve to increase the overload on your muscles, and thereby make them grow bigger. Other things being equal, *more* exercise, *more* sets, etc., make for *more* progress.

However, there's a point at which workout duration becomes *too* long, and results start to regress. At that point, you must reduce the length of your workouts considerably and adopt a new program. Then you formulate a new intensity drive in which, using your new routine, you gradually increase poundage and bring about sustained muscle growth.

The Carry-Along Principle

Perhaps this idea is best known as *specialization*, a technique that bodybuilders have been using successfully for many years. It has often been said that you cannot do justice to all your muscle groups all the time. That is why many men pay far more attention to one particular muscle group than to the others. They are concentrating on one area in order to bring that area up to par.

Say, for example, you had weak deltoids. It would make sense to start your workouts with *heavy press behind neck, seated dumbbell presses, lateral raises, and upright rows.* But you couldn't reasonably expect to use as many exercises for all other body parts; so you would merely "carry them along" with one basic movement that prevents the muscles from actually losing size and tone. This way, you don't push your whole body into a state of "overwork syndrome." You just push one particular area to a new plateau. When that's been achieved, you may want to resume a more balanced schedule. Alternatively, you may want to concentrate on some other part of your body.

It is not always feasible to achieve simultaneous gains in all areas; so this technique can be useful. Many top bodybuilders find it helpful. You will hear them say, "Yeah! I'm working my arms these days." All that means is that they are specializing on their arms by subjecting them to more exercises and sets with extra intensity, while minimizing the training for the rest of their body. It is *never* suggested, however, that you should eliminate *all* exercises for the rest of the body from your routine. If you just trained one muscle group exclusively, you wouldn't be gaining very much.

Holding Back

Cycling—or holding back for the sake of progression—is another method of derailing the sticking point. (Chapter 7 discussed this in greater detail.) In a sense, cycling—the process of gradually building up to peak performance—is an alternative to a lay-off. Even so, a complete rest from all training is a good idea once in a while.

At the beginning of a cycle, you should deliberately "hold back" in your efforts, so that you can later effect a steady progression. Instead of curling a 120 barbell all out for 5 sets of 10 reps, hold back on a couple of sets, or stop when you know that you could do a further one or two reps. There is no need to perform *more* exercises or *tougher* ones than you need to maintain an upward growth pattern. Ultimately, as you close in on your peaking period, you will be pushing all the buttons for utmost intensity. But while you are at the beginning or middle of a training cycle, you should be using your mind to control your energy output. Take pride in this control. Make your workouts *quietly optimistic.* Chaotic and panic-stricken struggles can lead only to staleness.

Going for a New Plateau

One thing's for sure: you cannot aim for and reach a new "high" in muscular development without first visualizing and then preparing for the task ahead. Your mind is the key to all significant progress. With iron-clad determination, you can achieve new and seemingly impossible results.

The first thing you have to do is to make sure that the body is in the proper condition to *authorize* a substantial gain. You must be tuned up, yet not overtrained. In other words, your body machinery must be used to heavy, tough training, but not to the point of near-exhaustion that puts you in a negative-growth phase. The base from which you "lift off" to a new plateau must be as solid as a rock. Your nervous system must not be shaky. Your food intake, supplementation, sleep, and rest must all be set for a new training push.

It's no use saying, "Tomorrow I will go for a new growth plateau." It doesn't work that way. You need at least 3–6 weeks of preparation. During this time, coax your muscles along, but be aware all along that you are holding back for the "push." Have no doubts that you will attain a new size and strength record. To doubt will be to fail. Be confident! Be absolutely *sure* that you will forge ahead, and you cannot possibly fail.

15

THE MUSCLE SLEEP

Snoozing for Size

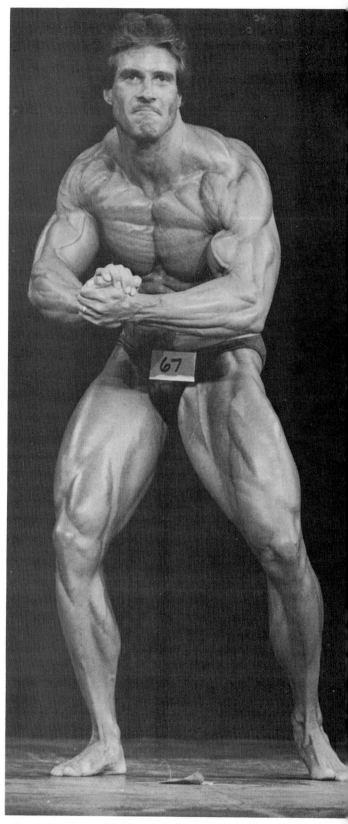

Bob Coburn, upcoming champion.

During World War II, the strategy and oratory of England's Winston Churchill united the British people against the tyranny of Hitler to a degree that no nation has been united since. Throughout the war, Churchill would stay awake and alert until three or four o'clock in the morning. His physical and mental endurance became a source of inspiration and wonderment to the allies, and even Adolf Hitler began to wonder whether the British prime minister was mortal. Eventually it was revealed that Churchill managed to stay alert into the wee hours of the morning because he took a quick nap in the afternoon.

There is little doubt that sleep is the most efficient way of maximizing recuperation. Experiments in Russia are said to have shown that several short naps during a 24-hour period can more than substitute for the uninterrupted seven or eight hours of sleep that most of us are accustomed to. The work and social system that we have chosen to live by is unfortunately not geared to this way of living. Few of us can work in three or four cat naps each day instead of the customary overnight slumber. People in

Latin countries enjoy an afternoon siesta, which recharges their batteries during the heat of the day, and so enables them to be active in the relative cool of the evening; but this is not the custom in most of Europe and North America.

The first person to use the term "muscle sleep" was another Britisher, photographer and bodybuilding writer Chris Lund. As a professional photographer, Chris was frequently on call at all hours of the day and night. The irregular sleep that this gave him was cutting into his training progress. Many a time he was not able to get to sleep until two or three in the morning, which left him pretty pooped when it came to his heavy-duty workout the following day. So, he would try and make up his lost sleep by taking forty winks during the lunch break after eating his midday meal. Amazingly, Lund found that even though he had missed several hours of sleep the previous night, he could make up this loss, or so it seemed, by grabbing a nap that lasted no more than 20 minutes. Muscle sleep had been born! It is the pause that refreshes.

The now middle-aged ballet dancer Rudolph Nureyev has for a long time been a source of amazement to his contemporaries. Performers of even half his age wonder how he manages to keep up such a high energy level. One of the answers is that the Russian dance genius sleeps for two hours after lunch.

Some people, though not all, seem to have the ability to sleep at odd times. I will never forget an athletic meeting in the USA, where the star high-jumper, a black man 6 feet 8 inches tall, was dominating the event. His leaps seemed to be charged with atomic energy as he gradually and systematically destroyed the opposition. After each jump he would get back into his sweat suit, top and bottom, and then he would nonchalantly roll over and fall asleep! At the time, I thought this was highly amusing. I was amazed at how a man, with tens of thousands of people watching him, could fall asleep when he wanted to; and upon waking, he needed little more than a shake of the head and a couple of stretches to ready himself for a further attempt at the high jump bar. Needless to say, he won the event outright.

The next time I saw an athlete sleeping in between physical exertions was on watching Serge Nubret train the last few weeks before he entered a NABBA Mr. Universe contest (which

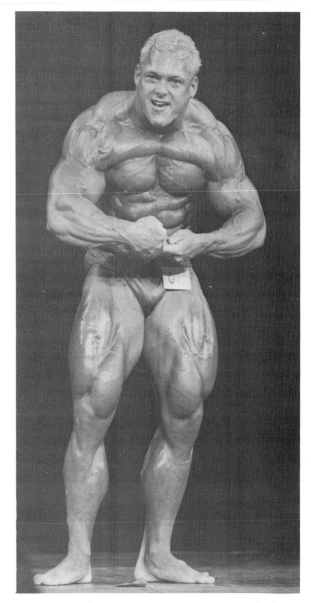

An unbelievable "Most Muscular" by Mr. America, Tim Belknap.

he won). After performing a dozen sets of high repetition bench presses, Serge maintained his supine position, closed his eyes, and dozed off for a couple of minutes. Later on, after resuming the workout, Nubret again fell asleep after completing a series of leg presses. I asked him the why's and wherefore's of his constant naps, and he explained to me that during his last few weeks of preparation he was on a very low carbohydrate diet, which gave him limited amounts of energy. He felt that the naps enabled him to "let go" totally and allowed his body to recharge itself for continuing the workout.

In all honesty, the muscle sleep is neither practical for everyone, nor is it necessarily recommended. I mention it for no other reason than that it *is* used, especially by pro bodybuilders during their last month before an important contest. For a short period, usually during the afternoon, they relax completely in order to maximize their post-workout recuperation.

If your work situation allows you the luxury of muscle sleep during a particularly grueling series of workouts, then some experimentation along these lines may help your progress.

At first, you may feel groggy after a 20-minute muscle sleep, and confused with regard to your surroundings or even the time of day. But when you get used to it, muscle-sleep will become a natural part of your day, and you will wake from it totally refreshed and ready to go. If you have had a full night's sleep, don't nap for more than 20 minutes; that would make your body lazy and sap your energy by taking you too far into the sleep cycle. Needless to say, the most effective muscle sleep will be one that you take in a darkened room with as little disturbing noise as possible.

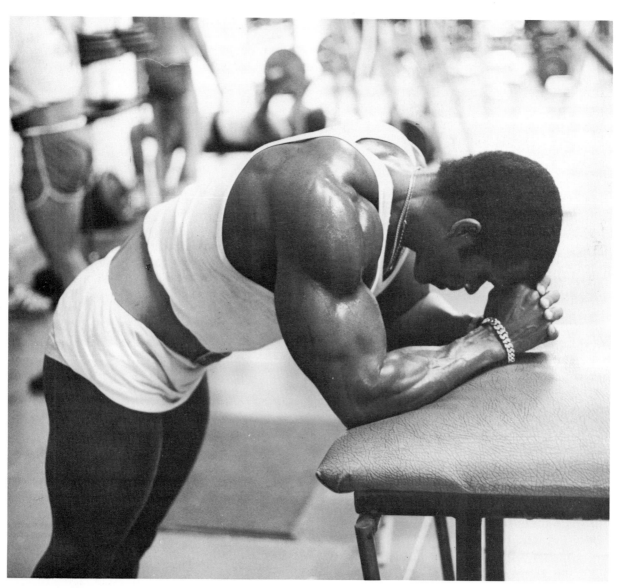

Serge Nubret takes a much-needed breather.

16
SHOULDERS
Building Impressive Barn-Door Width

Mike Mentzer's incredible delts.

Mother Nature seldom dishes out everything. In the case of shoulders . . . well, she either gives us narrow clavicles (the bone width) with plenty of cellular tissue to build big delts (shoulder muscles), or else we are given wide clavicles with a correspondingly poor allocation of muscle cells. Needless to say, we all want wide shoulders as well as trillions of muscle cells, so that we can really max-out our shoulder impressiveness.

The shoulders are a complex area. Unlike the knee joint, which is one-directional (it only goes up and down), the shoulder has a ball-and-socket type joint, which allows you to move your arm around in a circle with a very wide range of motions. In order to cope with this range, the shoulder muscles are divided into three separate "heads": the *anterior* (front), *medial* (side), and *posterior* (rear) deltoid.

No exercise *really* works all three sections at once, although there is some assistance from other parts of the shoulder, but it is practical to work one head at a time. The press behind neck works the side deltoid mainly, with some help from the rear head, whereas the bench press works the front deltoid with a little involvement from the side section—and, of course, the triceps and pecs.

Deltoid isolation exercises are used frequently. They include the alternate front dumbbell raise for the anterior (front) head, the lateral raise for the medial (side) head, and the bent-over flying movement for the posterior (rear) head.

Good as these isolation exercises are for hitting precise sections of the shoulder muscles, some kind of combination movement such as pressing is necessary for full deltoid development. The standard military press and the press behind neck are regulars among top bodybuilders. Other variations include dumbbell pressing, either together or in an alterna.ing fashion. These may be done either standing or sitting. Sitting enforces greater exercise strictness, so this will probably benefit your deltoid development more.

Upright rowing is another recommended shoulder movement which can really balloon out your delts. Of course, strands and pulleys, though limited in overall body application, also help shoulder development. You can perform lateral raises from a variety of angles with both types of apparatus, and there is a very good shoulder movement exclusive to the strandpuller: the back press!

The competitive bodybuilder should realize the importance of large, fully developed shoulders, because you cannot hide this area. Deltoids are seen from all angles—front, back,

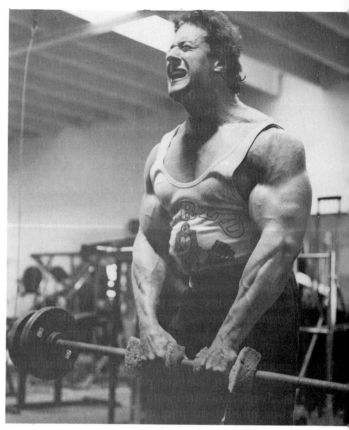

Upright rowing, demonstrated by Greg DeFerro. Note the sponges to aid gripping.

John Cardillo working the delts on a special shoulder machine.

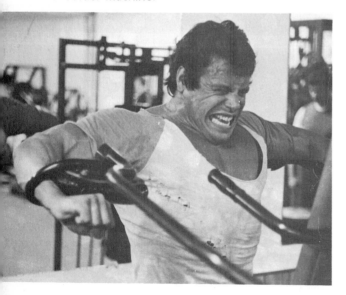

and sides. They are especially evident when you perform the double-biceps pose from the rear. To produce championship-quality shoulders, you need a routine that works all three deltoid heads. If on the other hand, your time is greatly limited and you can only perform one exercise for the shoulder region, I would suggest that this exercise be either the press behind neck or the alternate dumbbell press. Alternating with a see-saw action is usually preferable, since the mechanics of the movement dictate that you don't lean back, as you would tend to if you were pressing two dumbbells simultaneously. (By leaning back, the stress of the movement is thrown from the side deltoid head to the frontal area, so that you'll get thicker delts, but not wider ones.)

The tradition of mammoth shoulders has been with us for centuries. The ancient Greeks, for example, revered their wide-shouldered, athletic Adonis, and fiction rarely introduces us to a hero who is not broad-shouldered. To you, as an

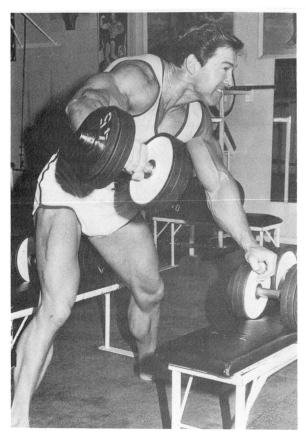

An unusual shoulder exercise. Scott gives it his all.

aspiring competitive bodybuilder, the shoulder muscles are all-important. You need them in virtually *every* pose, and when you are compared in the relaxed position, they are *everything*.

It is true that jackets and overcoats are invariably made with shoulder pads which give even the skinniest guy the appearance of shoulder width and development, but isn't it nice to be able to take off that jacket and still have that shoulder impressiveness?

Most comprehensive workouts will include two or three deltoid exercises. However, one should be aware of two facts:

1. Bench press and incline presses work the *frontal* deltoids very strongly.

2. Bent-over rowing exercises work the *rear* deltoids strongly.

Therefore, if you include some form of bench press and rowing exercise, then you don't necessarily have to include isolation exercises for the front and rear deltoids. Certainly, there is no need for the beginner or the man on a tight time schedule to do so.

Beginners should only perform one shoulder exercise: the press behind neck or the alternate dumbbell press.

Intermediates will find it best to perform one combination shoulder exercise (such as the seated press or the press behind neck) plus the bent-over flying movement and the lateral raise.

Advanced men, who will invariably be splitting their routine into two or more sections, will probably find the following most advantageous: two combination delt movements (such as press behind neck and upright rowing) followed by alternate forward dumbbell raise, lateral raise, and bent-over flying.

Here are some of the best shoulder exercises I have ever found. I will explain how they should be performed. Although there is more than one way to skin the proverbial cat, I believe my way is the best—in some cases, only by a small margin. The press behind neck exercise, for example, can very effectively be performed standing up, especially if the weight is taken from squat stands; but I have specified that it be performed sitting down. This makes it a slightly more effective movement, but that is not to say that you should not experiment. Bear in mind, too, that an *inferior* exercise may prove an effective substitute for a really fine movement, merely because your muscles (and mind) crave a change. A change can work wonders.

Lance Dreher—laterals on a pulley for side deltoids.

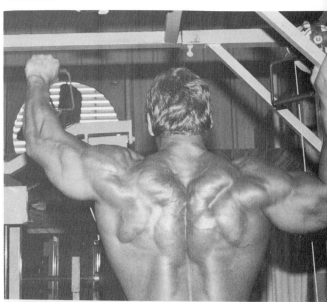

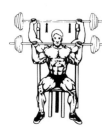

Press Behind Neck
Side Deltoid (6–12 reps each set)

Sitting down on a special upright bench with supports, take a loaded barbell, with your hand spacing sufficiently wide that when your upper arms are parallel to the floor, your forearms are in a vertical position. Lower the weight as far as possible behind the neck, and immediately raise when it touches your trapezius. Do *not* bounce the bar from your shoulders. Keep your elbows as far back as possible throughout the movement. Lock out the elbows as the arms extend overhead, but do not hold the position. Continue pressing up and down, rhythmically without any pause.

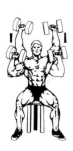

Alternate Dumbbell Press
Side Deltoid (8–12 reps each set)

Work in sitting position, back flat. Start the movement with a pair of dumbbells held at the shoulders, palms of the hands facing inwards or forward. Hold elbows back to maintain stress on side deltoids. Start with your weakest hand, and alternately press first one dumbbell, then the other, in a see-saw fashion. Lock out the arm each time you press the weight, but do not maintain the straight arm position; as soon as your arm straightens, lower it, and continue the exercise with no pauses whatsoever.

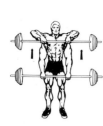

Upright Rowing
Front and Side Deltoids (8–15 reps each set)

Use a fairly wide grip. The wider the grip, the more stress is put on the side deltoid. A narrow grip will put more effort on the frontal deltoid and the trapezius. Always straighten the arms at the bottom of the exercise, and start your pull slowly, gathering momentum as the weight rises to your chin area. Keep the up-down movement rhythmic. Maintain an upright stance with feet comfortably apart, (12–15 inches). As the bar rises, try to keep your elbows as high as possible.

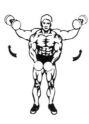

Lateral Raise
Side Deltoids (8–12 reps each set)

A thousand and one ways to perform this exercise, all with one purpose: to throw the stress onto the side deltoids. (Everyone wants more shoulder width!) Perform this exercise seated on the end of a bench. Feet flat on the floor together, ankles touching. Arms must be bent to almost "right angles" to throw stress on the all-important (that width again!) lateral deltoids. Raise the weights, from the arms-straight-at-sides position to level with your head, and immediately lower. Keep palms facing downwards throughout. At time of extreme effort, try and lean forward "into" the exercise, rather than backwards (which will again put stress on the powerful front deltoids).

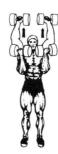

The Arnold Press
Side and Front Deltoids (10–15 reps each set)

This exercise is a pure bodybuilding movement. The mechanics involved are not at all in line with the accepted or "natural" way to lift a particular weight overhead, but the movement does build muscle. Reportedly, the exercise was first used in the "golden age" of bodybuilding, the sixties muscle-beach scene. It was a favorite with Larry Scott, who is said to have explained it to the great Arnold Schwarzenegger. Arnold then used it so successfully that it became known as the "Arnold Press."

Begin this movement by holding a pair of dumbbells as you would at the top of a dumbbell curl. From this somewhat irregular position, press the dumbbells upward while rotating the thumbs inward. Do *not* lock out the arms at the conclusion of the part press, part lateral-raise exercise, but continue the up-down movement without pause to exhaust the deltoids fully.

Bent Over Flying
Rear Deltoid (10–15 reps each set)

This very important exercise is one of the few to work the rear shoulder region almost exclusively. Full development in the rear delts is a must in today's competitive arena, because anything less than maximum posterior delt size will leave all back poses up for criticism. The back deltoids also contribute to side-view thickness and counteract any round shoulder appearance you may have.

Sit on the end of an exercise bench with your knees and feet together. Lean forward until your chest touches your thighs. Raise your heels off the floor so that your thighs and chest are locked together, supported by your toes on the ground.

Holding a pair of light dumbbells, raise your arms out sideways, palms facing each other, until the weights are as high as you can get them. The arm should be unlocked (not straight) to alleviate pressure on the elbows. Always start this movement slowly, forcing your rear deltoids to work strongly to build up momentum during the last 12 inches before the conclusion of the raising motion. If you start off quickly from the hang position, you minimize the rear deltoid involvement and kill the main usefulness of the exercise.

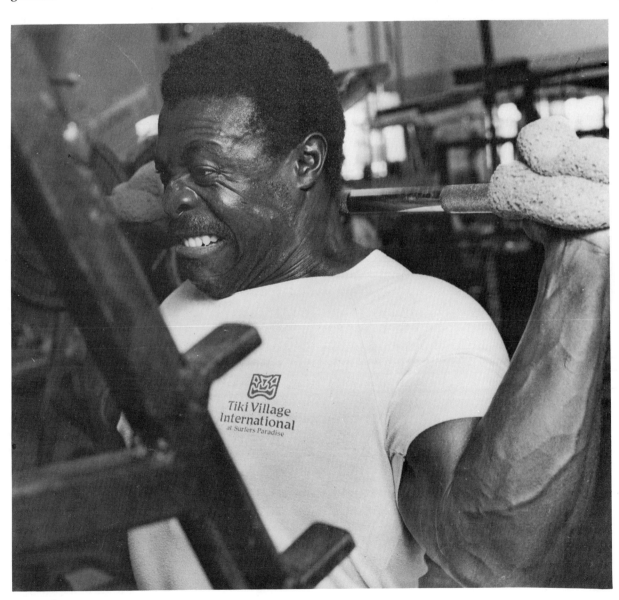

Roy Callendar. He has deltoids par excellence.
And here's why.

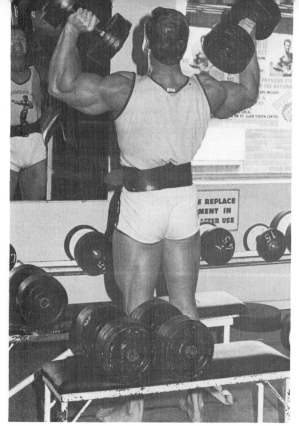

Larry Scott, considered to be one of the most intelligent trainers.

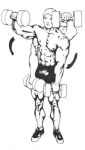

Alternate Dumbbell Front Raise
Front Deltoid (10–15 reps each set)

Hold a pair of dumbbells while in the standing position. Raise one hand directly forward until well above your eyeline, and then as it is lowered, raise the other hand. Continue this see-saw motion without pausing in any position. Do not lift both dumbbells out in front at the same time, because this would causes the torso to adjust the balance by leaning backwards, thus negating some of the stress on the front deltoids.

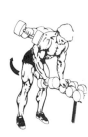

Single Arm Lateral Raise with Dumbbell
Side Deltoids (8–15 reps each set)

A great favorite with Boyer Coe and Larry Scott. The beauty of this exercise is that there is little stress on the lower back (which can cause discomfort) and you can lock yourself into a specific position, thereby avoiding all possibility of cheating.

Place your left arm on a suitable support (about 30 inches high). Most trainers use a dumbbell rack or low table. With your legs apart, hold a dumbbell in your right hand. Adopt a comfortable position with your torso bent forward at an angle of 70–80 degrees. Raise the dumbbell out to the side, keeping the palm of your hand facing downwards. Concentrate on making the shoulder muscle lift the weight (the arm should be unlocked but not excessively bent). Don't start this exercise with maximum thrust, otherwise you just lift the bell with momentum.

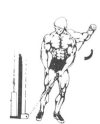

Back Press with Strands
Side Deltoids (15–25 reps each set)

Start by holding a set of strands behind your back, palms facing forward, elbows tight in at your sides. Press out the arms to a straight crucifix position. As soon as the arms straighten, return them to the original position and repeat the process.

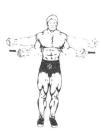

Seated Dumbbell Press
Side Deltoid (6–12 reps each set)

While seated, hold two dumbbells at the shoulders. Keep your back straight and your head up. Press both dumbbells simultaneously to the overhead position. Do not lean back during the exercise. Lower and repeat with a steady rhythm.

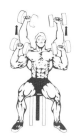

Lateral Raise with Strands or Pulleys
Side Deltoids (15–25 reps each set)

A fine finishing or pumping exercise to conclude your deltoid workout. You can use two pairs of strands, one hooked under each foot (or use low pulleys if you train in a well-equipped gym). Raise and lower your arms at equal speed without any pause. Hold your torso slightly bent forward in order to put stress exclusively on lateral head. Make this a continuous tension movement by keeping continuous pressure on the deltoids.

17
CHEST
Gaining New Pectoral Impressiveness

One of the greatest of all: Serge Nubret's chest.

Men like Franco Columbu and Serge Nubret get an enormous amount of pectoral development from the bench press. In fact, Nubret does no other pectoral exercise, except just before an important contest.

Vince Gironda says the regular bench press is 90 percent front deltoid, but when I was at Gironda's gym in North Hollywood, he and Erik Estrada were doing set after set of bench presses. The only difference was that they were lowering the bar to their neck instead of their pectorals.

"Vince, I thought you were against the bench press?" Vince seemed to take mild enjoyment from my shock at seeing him pump out rep after rep. "Hell, Kennedy, this is no bench press. We call this a *neck* press!"

The bench press is really a pretty remarkable exercise. It works for most people. Perhaps it gives the most gain to those who have a fairly shallow rib cage. With them, the bar has a great distance to travel and thus effects a great stretch of the pectorals, while a barrel-chested person, due to the size of his chest, may not be able to lower the bar very far, but that is not always the case. Reg Park had a pretty thick rib cage and still got a great deal from the bench press. And getting back to Gironda: even if you do have a thick or deep chest, you can always increase the *stretch* by lowering the bar to your neck. (No bouncing, though!) Man being ever the inventor, there is also a cambered bar on the market now which allows even the most deep-chested of men to get a full and complete stretch of the pectoral muscles.

The beauty of the bench press is that it is performed from a very comfortable and stable position—lying on your back, face up. After you get used to it, you do not have to concern yourself with balance or performance difficulty. As a result, and because the belly of the pectorals and triceps is involved, your strength and development grow when you practice the bench press regularly.

Many people think I am against the bench press, that I have an ongoing vendetta against this movement. What I am against is the abuse of the exercise. Happily, this is not so widespread today, but in the sixties and seventies, some bodybuilders were spending up to two-thirds of their workouts bench pressing! As a result, we saw bodybuilders with balloons instead of pectorals. What made matters worse was that these men were not giving enough time to their shoulder training, so the rest of them didn't have the proportions to complement their pectorals. They had no delts, no width. In fact, they looked like a deformed species, even though they undoubtedly felt like heroes. At the very least, big pecs should be accompanied by big deltoids.

Although the bench press can build a pretty good all-round chest, one should be aware of the other chest exercises that can help to balance your chest development. The bench press may not do it all for you. In fact, it probably won't. You will be rewarded, however, if you vary the width of your hand spacing when you bench press. A wide hand spacing puts the exercise stress on the outer part of the pectoral. A medium grip will hit the middle part of the chest, and a narrow grip will develop the inner pectorals. (Of course, the triceps are also strongly activated by narrow-grip bench presses.)

The bench press, King of Exercises, performed by Bronston Austin, Jr.

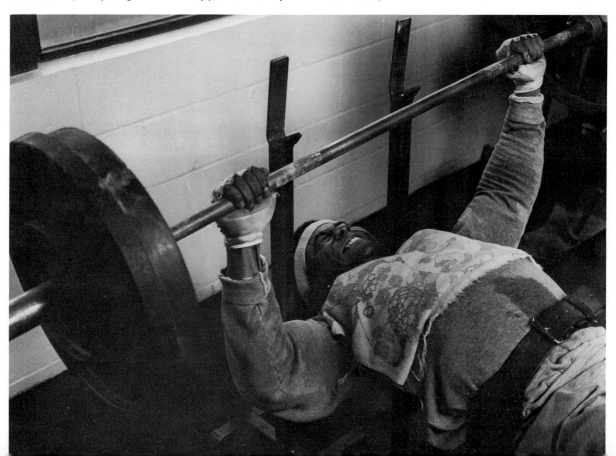

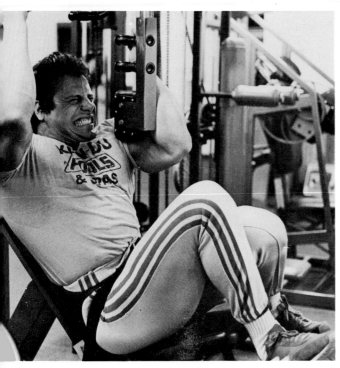

John Cardillo works his chest one side at a time, on Nautilus.

Watch It!

As with other exercises, you must try to forget the aspect of hoisting up the weight. Bouncing, twisting, lifting the hips from the bench, in order to get the weight up is *not* the best way to build great pecs. On the contrary, you should use the weight correctly as a tool to achieve your goal. Here is Arnold Schwarzenegger's thinking on this subject: "The trick to bodybuilding is to put an overload on your muscles. The secret is not so much to get the weight up as it is to push up a heavy weight with the *isolated* strength of the muscles you are trying to train."

One of the greatest errors when chest training, according to expert Bill Reynolds, is lack of concentration. It's so important to flex the pectoral muscles throughout the movements.

Another mistake is to follow someone else's routine set for set without concern for the particular needs of your own body.

Finally, always remember to stretch the pectorals fully. After your first warm-up sets, you can really bring out the arms and fully extend the motion affecting the pectorals. In most cases, the use of dumbbells allows for more of a stretch than the use of barbells.

As you lower the weight, you activate whatever area is in line with the bar. If you lower the bar to your lower chest, you will work the lower chest. Bring the weight to the middle of your pecs, and that is where you will stimulate most growth. Lower the bar to the upper chest for . . . right! . . . upper pec development. Naturally, there is some spillover effect. Even though you are working for development in one area, bear in mind other parts of the pectorals will also be stimulated.

When sculpting your pectorals, bear in mind that incline presses with a barbell or dumbbells will work the upper chest. Flyes work the outer pecs (some inner development is achieved when the dumbbells are brought together, but at this point the resistance is minimal). Regular dips involve the lower pectorals, but if the dipping bars are moved out to 28–34 inches (taller people need wider bars), then you will work the upper and outer area of the pectorals.

Pullovers help the rib cage, but do not expect any dramatic rib cage expansion. Expansion will eventually take place, but only within the framework of your skeletal genetics.

Dumbbell presses by Bronston Austin, Jr.

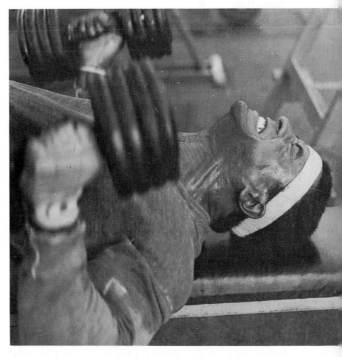

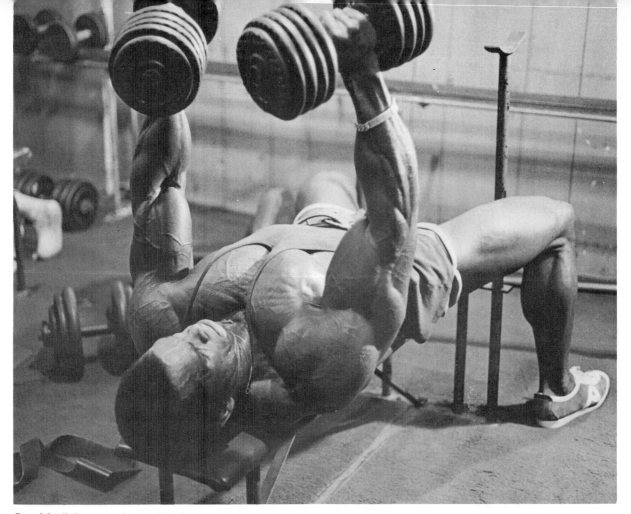

Dumbbell flyes performed Nubret-style.

Now to the exercises.

Bench Press
Overall Pectoral Area
(5–15 reps each set)

Known as the King of Exercises, the bench press can be tailored to any part of the pectoral muscles. If the exercise is to benefit the upper chest, then lower the bar to the neck. Lower the bar to the mid-pectorals, and that is where the effect will be felt. Narrow-grip bench presses (10 inches) will activate the inner pecs. The outer chest is worked with a wide hand spacing. You can tailor the bench press to pinpoint any area for muscle development by choosing the right grip width and bar groove.

The standard way of performing the bench press is to take a grip, with your thumbs about 3 feet (90 cm) apart, which allows the forearms to be vertical when the upper arms are parallel to the floor.

Start while lying face up on a bench. Take a balanced hand placing, using the thumbs-under-the-bar grip (not essential). Lower the weight from the arms-straight position to the pectorals. Touch the bar lightly to the chest (no bouncing) and press upwards. Keep your elbows under the bar, and don't allow them to come close to the body.

Beginners may find that the bar starts to fall either forwards or backwards, or that the weight is rising unevenly because one arm is stronger than the other. Time and practice will cure these mild upheavals. After a few weeks, you won't even have to think about balancing the weight or lowering it without wobbling because you will have then developed a perfect groove.

When you lower the bar to the chest, don't allow it to drop! Always control its descent deliberately, especially so if it is a heavy weight. Control its downward path, and you are assured of a positive upward movement.

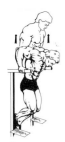

Parallel Bar Dips
(8–20 reps each set)

A wonderful chest movement, especially if the bars are set fairly wide apart (28–34 inches, or 70–85 cm). Narrow-set parallel bars will promote more triceps activity, but will still work the lower and outer pectorals. Wider-set parallel bars will benefit the upper outer part of the chest. The visual impact of this development will be to make you look wide in the upper torso and shoulders.

When working the chest on the dip bars, place your legs in front of your body, keep your head down (chin on chest) and elbows well out to the sides. Lower yourself as far down as possible and lock out the elbows as you straighten up.

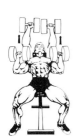

Incline Dumbbell Bench Press
Upper Chest (8–12 reps each set)

Start by lying on an incline bench set at a 35–40 degree angle. (More than 40 degrees will put too much emphasis on front deltoids.) Press the dumbbells simultaneously straight upwards, lock out the elbows, and immediately lower the weights to the starting position. Keep the up-down movement going without pause. Palms should be facing forward throughout the exercise.

Incline dumbbell presses by John Cardillo.

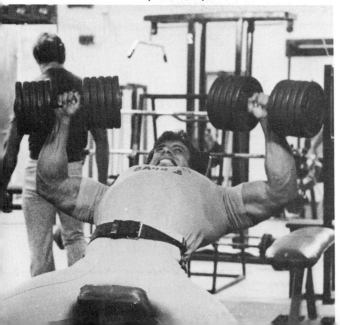

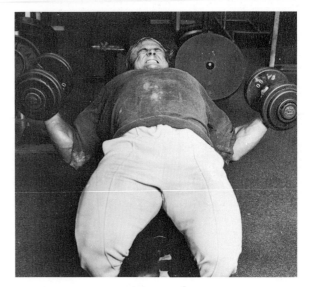

Tom Platz—chest training.

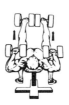

Flat Bench Press with Dumbbells
Mid-Chest Area (6–12 reps)

Lie on your back and hold two dumbbells with your arms fully extended at right angles to the floor. Lower both dumbbells to the chest and immediately press them up again to their original position. Do not bounce the weights from the chest. Keep your elbows out from the body during the movement.

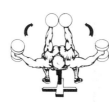

Supine Flying
Outer Pectorals (10–12 reps each set)

Years ago this exercise was done very rigidly with light weights on the floor. Very light dumbbells were used, since the experts of the day insisted that the arms be fixed in an elbows-locked, straight position. Today we still insist on a fixed position, but one in which the arms are bent as though they were in a plaster cast. This takes the strain off the elbow joint, allows more weight to be used, gives you greater dumbbell control and . . . yes, bigger chest muscles!

While lying face up on a bench, with your feet planted firmly on the ground, lower and raise the dumbbells out to the side. Really *go* for the stretch once your muscles are warmed up. Keep arms "locked" in the unlocked position.

97

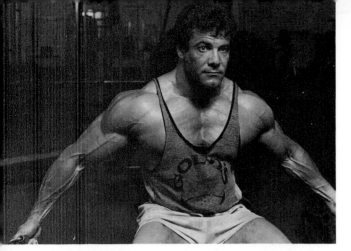

Canada's Reid Schindle. The Gentle Giant performs crossovers from a low angle.

Incline Flyes
Upper and Outer Chest (8–12 reps)

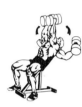

Adopt a secure position on an inclined bench (a 30–40 degree angle is best). Hold up a pair of light dumbbells, then allow your arms to lower slowly out to the sides. Keep elbows slightly bent throughout the exercise. Raise and lower slowly, keeping the weights under control as each repetition stretches the chest.

Decline Bench Press with Dumbbells
Lower Chest (8–12 reps)

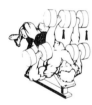

Lie on a declined bench as shown. Press up and then lower both dumbbells simultaneously, as you would in the regular flat bench dumbbell bench press. Keep your elbows as far out (sideways) from the body as possible.

Samir Bannout performing crossover pulleys.

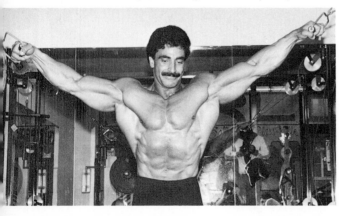

Incline Barbell Bench Press
Upper Chest (8–12 reps)

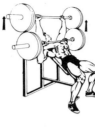

Take a loaded barbell while in an incline position on a secure bench. Lower it slowly to the upper chest, elbows out to the side, and then push it to the arms-straight position. Lower and repeat.

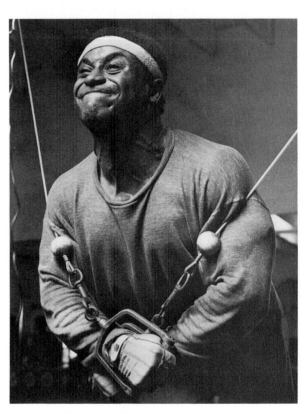

Bronston Austin, Jr. likes crossover pulley work for cutting up his chest.

Cable Crossovers
Overall Chest (10–15 reps)

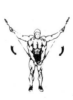

This is a specialized exercise. Cable crossover machines are expensive, but most modern gyms do have them. Holding the cable handles, bend your arm slightly at the elbow and bring your hands together in front of your chest or hips. Try and concentrate the action onto the chest area. Keep the arms "locked" in a slightly bent position throughout the exercise.

18
ABDOMINAL TRAINING
Wasting Away for Midsection Impressiveness

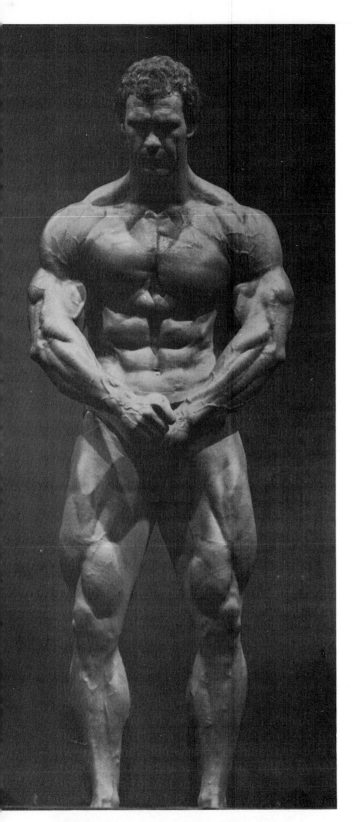

Bodybuilding sensation Scott Wilson has the waistline of a true champion.

Mike Mentzer said it: "It is best never to allow enough fat to accumulate so the abs become memories."

Whatever fat starts to settle around the midsection is going to have to be removed one day, which usually means that you will have to put yourself into a negative calorie balance for a considerable period. This will, of course, tend to hold back or diminish overall muscle gains. Far better to keep your abs throughout your training career, so that when contest time comes around you will only require minimal dieting.

Many beginners are puzzled as to whether or not one can change the shape or evenness of the ab muscles. I agree that a set of "line-up" abs running across the tummy in even rows is most impressive, but few people actually possess this, not even the great Steve Reeves. Unfortunately, *no* amount of exercise will change the placement of your ab muscles. If they are uneven now, then that is how they will stay for life.

Famous bodybuilders who do have even rows of abdominals include Mohamed Makkawy, Leo Robert, Dennis Tinerino, and Samir Bannout. There are, of course, others whom you will see in the various bodybuilding books and

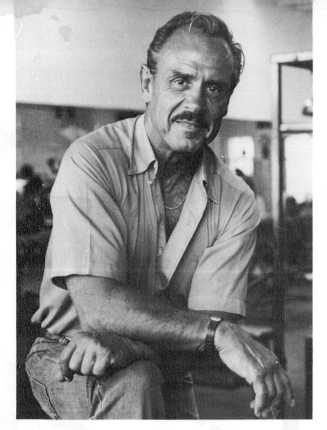

The "boss," Zabo Koszewski—a very real part of World's Gym. Holder of more "best ab" titles than anyone else.

For many years bodybuilders trained their abs with very high repetitions. This practice is frowned upon by many of the modern bodybuilders, yet there is still a core of followers of the high-rep theory. Bill Pearl, when training for a contest or exhibition, has been known to perform hundreds of reps for the waist. Frank Zane performs sets of 200 reps. Irvin Koszewski trains his waist by the clock: 30 minutes per set at minimum. In his heyday, he never did less than 1,000 repetitions.

Vince Gironda was the first who publicly called for rep moderation. "The abs are just another muscle group, super-high reps are not needed," said the Iron Guru. Mike Mentzer followed up by advocating a system of no more than 12–15 reps for abdominal movements.

It is obvious that both methods work, but in this day of rush and haste, time saving is often an important factor. Why do more when you can get the same results by doing less?

Actually, the abdominal area is very sensitive to heavy exercise, and high-intensity effort is suitable only for the more rugged individuals. If the average man were to go all-out with heavy reps in his abdominal exercises, this could stop his overall gains in development. The midsection fascia is a center of the body's nervous pathways. By overworking it, you will shock your

Look at the wonderful midsection of Samir Bannout.

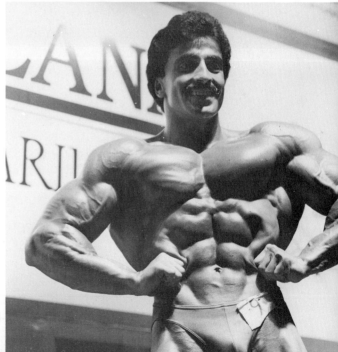

magazines. However, it is no great sin to have uneven layers of waist musculature. Mr. Abs himself, Irvin "Zabo" Koszewski, had uneven abdominals. Yet he won just about every "best abs" contest he entered until he was well past forty years of age. Everybody, but everybody, wanted abs like Irvin's.

Among the uninitiated, it is commonly thought that one can get the abdominal muscles to show by performing a few sets of situps or leg raises every day. This is not true. If there is a covering of fat around the waistline, then the direct abdominal exercise will only build the muscle density *under* the fat. Invariably, this is *not* enough to get them to show up as impressively as one would like. In fact, it is quite likely that they won't show up at all.

The answer, then, is diet. Your nutritional intake must be revised to a new, lower calorie consumption. Remember that if you took a year or two to put the fat on your waist, you are not likely to remove it with a couple of weeks dieting. A very determined and sometimes lengthy period of dieting is often required.

entire system, which may cause a temporary shutdown of the growth process.

My own thoughts run to performing moderately high repetitions for abs—around 15–30 per set. You will find out by trial and error what appears to work best for you. In any case, it is not a good idea to do a great deal of abdominal exercising late at night. Such overstimulation could lead to a sleepless night—a situation that's not relished by the hopeful champion.

For those who are carrying excess baggage (fat) around their waistline, it is a biological fact that 3,500 calories equal one pound of fat. Accordingly, if you wish to lose one pound of fat every week, you would have to cut 500 calories per day from your normal diet. It is easy to lose one pound a week by making small food sacrifices here and there.

Today, there are literally thousands of bodybuilders who have superb abdominal muscles. This contrasts greatly with the physique stars of yesteryear. Only a handful of them had outstanding midsections.

Have you noticed, when looking at some of the muscle publications, that many bodybuilders seem to have oversized, chunky, and noticeably bloated stomach muscles? This is usually caused by the taking of artificial anabolic steroids, often in large uncontrolled quantities.

An unaesthetic midsection bloat does not win over a contest audience or the judges. If your abdominals look a little bloated as a contest date is zooming up, it may be a good idea to cease all direct abdominal work during the last ten days. You can keep them toned by your posing practice, which you will undoubtedly pursue with vigor as the show date approaches. Without heavy exercise, the edema (bloat) should vanish and make your waistline look much trimmer to the all-important judging panel.

I have seen some pretty remarkable things happen to bodybuilders, and I always admire

Tom Platz checks his incredible abs in the mirror.

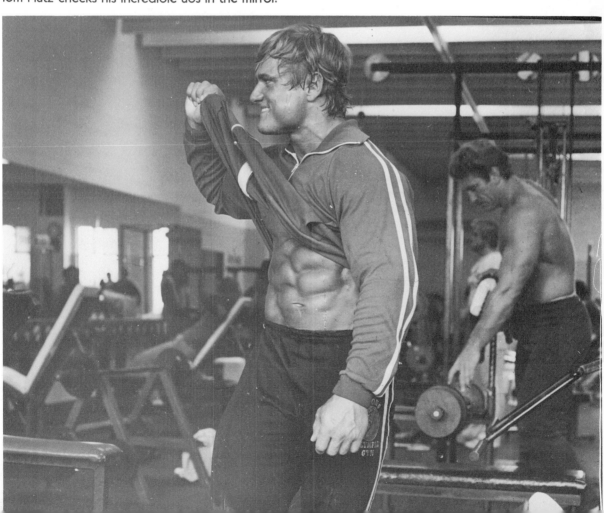

those who can combine exercise and diet to bring out their abdominals, especially when they manage to bring them out from nowhere (I should say from behind a wall of flab). In some cases, this happens over and over again. Yet, one should not make a habit of losing one's abs at the end of each summer only to blitz off the flab the following spring.

Special care should be taken not to stretch the abdominal wall. This can happen through overindulging in beer (large amount at one sitting) or through performing heavy squats (don't they call them gut-bustin' squats?) without wearing a strong leather belt, or even through pushing your tummy out, as some guys are inclined to do for a joke. Look at the abdominal wall as a coil spring. Pull it out a certain distance and let go. It zips back into the coiled position. But pull it out a greater distance and the strain is too much for the metal. It doesn't spring back when you let it go. Nothing you can do will make it zip back.

There are scores of different midsection exercises, and they all work to a degree. Here are some of the best I have found in my travels.

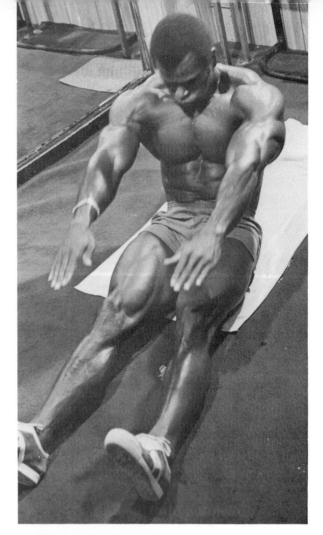

Sit-ups—Serge Nubret style.

Serge Nubret performs broomstick twists for his waistline.

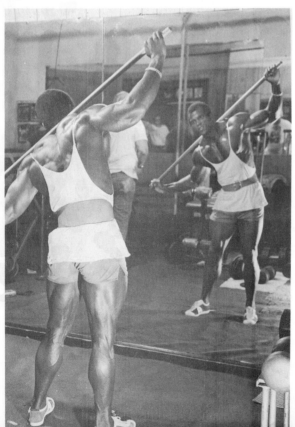

 Incline Twisting Sit-ups
Lying back on an incline board set at any angle you choose (the steeper the angle the lower the part of the waist worked). Your feet should be held to the board with a strap (or bar under which the feet fit). Place your hands behind your head and curl upwards. Keep the knees slightly bent throughout the movement.

Roman Chair Sit-ups
You need a Roman chair to anchor your legs in position and allow the trunk to sink below parallel, thus working the abdominal region to a greater degree. Perform this with a steady rhythm and no bouncing. This is the favorite exercise of Irvin "Zabo" Koszewski, who has won more "best abdominals" awards than any other bodybuilder.

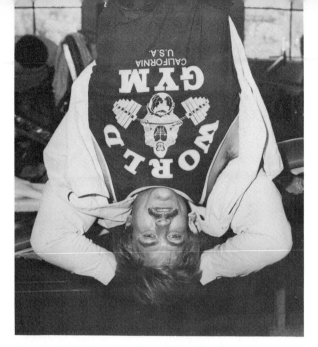

Roger Callard works his waist using inversion boots.

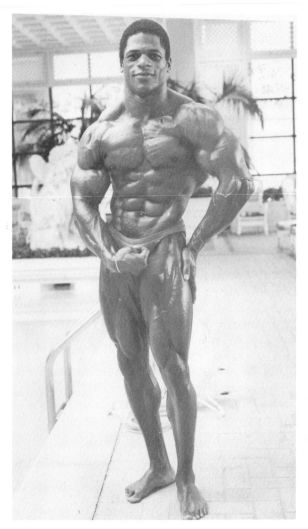

Hanging Leg Raise

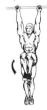

Hang from an overhead horizontal bar, with your arms about 30 inches (75 cm) apart. Keeping your legs straight, raise them until they are just past the parallel-to-floor position; then lower and repeat. Try not to let the body build up a swinging motion. This exercise works the very important lower abdominal region, right down to the groin.

For those who are unable to perform this exercise with straight legs, start off with the knees bent. Tuck your knees into the waist at each repetition, and point your toes downwards. Start the raise slowly, with positively no swinging. After a few weeks you will be able to graduate to the straight-leg style.

Always in shape, and never without his super sharp abdominals: Mr. America, Mr. Universe, Tony Pearson.

Tom Platz. Supine knee raises.

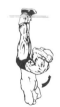

Inversion Boot Sit-ups

An excellent movement for the lower tummy area. Using a pair of inversion or gravity boots, hang from a strongly supported horizontal bar. Curl upwards in an upside-down sit-up, lower slowly, and repeat.

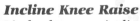

Incline Knee Raise

Lie back on an inclined bench (the angle can be varied) and secure your position by holding on at a suitable place. Raise the legs, bending the knees as they rise. Lower to the straight-leg position slowly, and repeat.

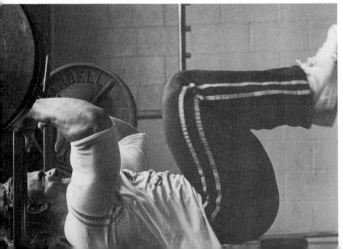

103

19
PUTTING YOUR BACK INTO IT
Working the Lats and Traps

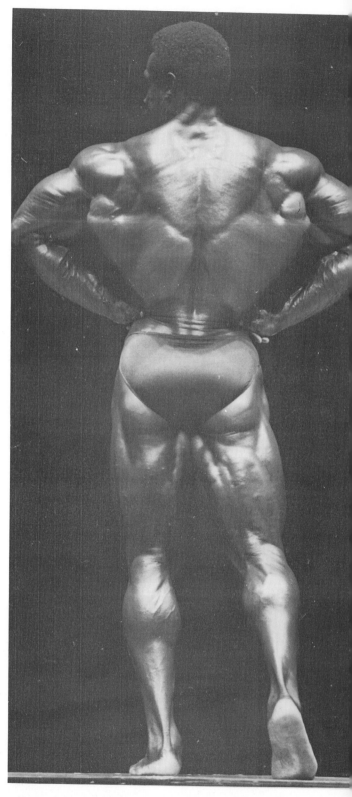

Look at the perfectly proportioned back of Roy Callendar.

Nature has arranged the human body in such a way that the two biggest muscles of the back—the lats (latissimus dorsi) and the traps (trapezius)—can actually be seen, not only from the back, which one would expect, but also from the front. This is especially true when these two major back muscles are fully developed. The other area which concerns the bodybuilder is the lower back: the two columns of lumbar region, the erector spinae. These are very powerful muscles which, when fully developed, create an impression of strength and virility.

Beautifully sculpted backs, as we are used to seeing them today, just were not around fifty years ago. True, the strongmen of the times did have thickness and mass, but the enormous, excessively tapered backs of our current era are a relatively new phenomenon.

The supreme back of the 40's belonged to John Carl Grimek, followed by the perfectly proportioned back of the Hercules of the screen, Steve Reeves. This man had an absolutely amazing back, developed in every facet. His traps reached up into his column-like neck. He had wide flaring lats, and his lumbar region was also superb. Little wonder Reeves won every top title of his era.

Reg Park took back development a step further. A new massiveness was born in the 50's, and for more than a decade Reg was ahead of the pack. Like Reeves, he had width and taper, but with an added dimension: Herculean thickness!

In the late 60's and 70's, two bodybuilders vied for the top titles: Sergio Oliva and Arnold Schwarzenegger. Both had amazing backs. Sergio had the edge over Arnold when it came to V-shape (will his phenomenal taper ever be equalled?), but Arnold had it over Sergio with regard to thickness and etched-in muscularity.

Today we have a host of stars with incredible back development. Lance Dreher must have the most massive of all. He has both width and thickness. Tony Pearson appears to possess the widest back of the current crop; and for perfect all-round shape and proportion and with the added attraction of size, Chris Dickerson is hard to fault.

Many people worry that the development of the trapezius will detract from the visual width of the physique. This is not so. What detracts from the visual width of the body is underdeveloped shoulders and wide waist and hips. The only time one should refrain from performing specific trapezius exercises is when one has inherited a short neck. Heavy trap development will give the short-necked bodybuilder an unattractive hunchiness.

One of the most spectacular traps that I have seen belongs to Serge Nubret (who incidentally seldom works them directly). Because of his superbly small waistline and hips, and even though he has huge traps, Nubret looks extremely wide in the shoulders.

The lats are the biggest muscles of the back. They are "wings" that can be seen from the front under the arms. There are two ways to approach lat building. First, the scapulas (shoulder blades) must be stretched out. This is done with wide-grip chins, either in front or behind the neck, or by doing the lat spread pose. Then thickness must be built in the area, usually by performing one or more of the various bent-over rowing movements.

As a result of inherited traits, some men possess high lats and others low lats. The vast majority of us are somewhere in between. It is generally accepted that a man with high lat de-velopment (like Johnny Fuller) should perform plenty of rowing movements, pulling the bar into the waist to work the belly of the muscle, whereas a low-lat individual (like Franco Columbu) requires no further development in the bottom regions and could concentrate on stretching out the upper areas with wide-grip chins. Natural shape or type cannot be totally turned around, of course, but some changes can be accomplished.

I feel that it is important for most bodybuilders to train the lats for width and thickness, which means that they should make a point of doing at least two lat exercises (one stretching movement and one rowing movement) each back workout. The question has been raised as to which is the superior exercise for pulling out the lats: the wide-grip chin, or the wide-grip lat-machine pulldown. Theoretically, the lat machine wins, because the pulldown motion can be extensively controlled, in that you can bring the bar way down below the shoulder level if

Low pulley rowing, as done by Serge Nubret, Mr. Universe.

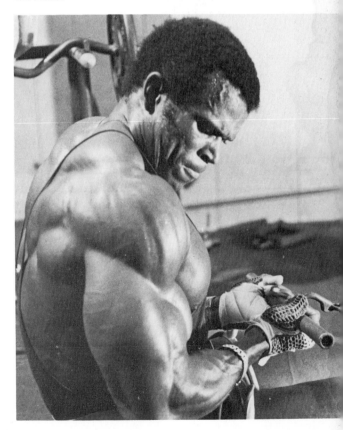

you wish (by adding to the range of resistance). Also, the lat machine permits a greater variety of reps with very little inconvenience. If you wanted to perform numerous sets of 30 reps, for example, you would have to use a lat machine—unless you are a superman.

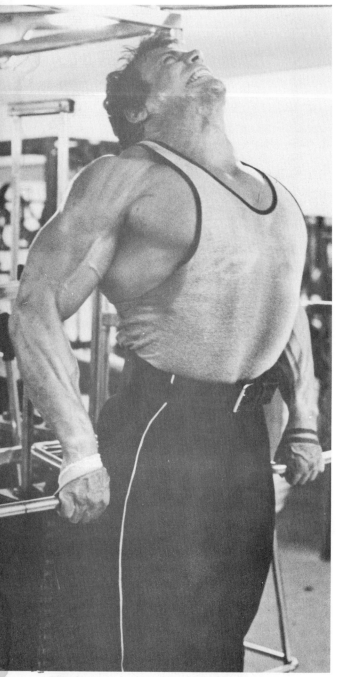

Working the traps with shrugs—Canada's John Cardillo.

Ironically, theory isn't always the winner. There is no doubt that the chin where the body is pulled up to the bar does confer some benefit that the pulldown motion does not. This is my feeling (and apparently that of most top bodybuilders). Hardly a scientific conclusion, I admit, yet it appears to be correct, at least until disproven.

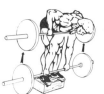

Bent-over Rowing

This is one of the most popular exercises for putting some meat on your lats. Grab a barbell with hands about 24 inches (60 cm) apart. Bend your knees slightly, and keep your head as high as possible while bending your torso parallel to the floor. Keep your lower back flat, your seat stuck outwards, and pull up vigorously on the bar. Pull it into the tummy, not the chest. Lower it until your arms are completely stretched, and more. Do not rest weight on floor until set is completed. Pull up, and repeat.

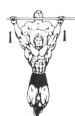

Low Pulley Rowing

Perform this movement with a long cable machine. Secure your feet against the apparatus, and pull the cable handles horizontally into your midsection. Hold for a second and slowly allow your arms to straighten and ultimately stretch your lats. Pull in again, and repeat. Aim to maximize that stretch as the arms straighten.

Wide-Grip Chin

Grasp an overhead bar using an overgrip (palms down) at least a foot wider than your shoulders on either side. (If your shoulders are 2 feet (60 cm) across, take a grip about 4 feet (120 cm) wide.) Pull upwards, keeping your elbows back throughout the movement. You may pull up so that the bar is either in front or behind your neck. That choice is entirely up to you. Some bodybuilders like to change around for variety, but it would not be correct to say that one form is superior to the other. Lower until your arms are straight, and repeat.

Once you can perform 12–15 reps, it is a good idea to attach added weight with the help of a weight belt. After that, you can build up your reps again.

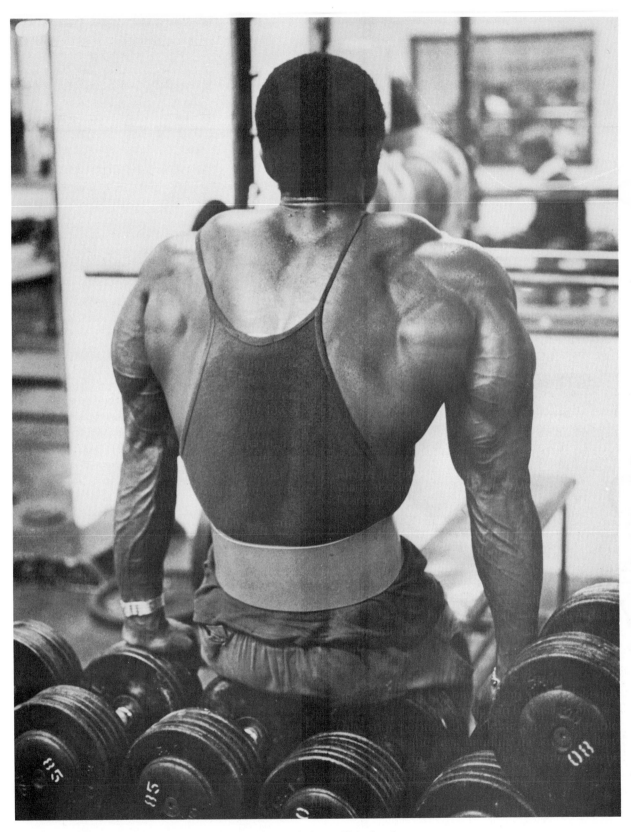

What a V-shape! Serge Nubret is the owner of this incredible back.

T-Bar Rows

This movement, primarily for the belly of the latissimus, is performed on a special apparatus. The movement is almost identical to the bent-over barbell rowing motion, except that one end of your lever bar is anchored to the floor. As a result of this, there may be less strain on the lower back.

Single-Arm Dumbbell Rowing

Another "total" lat exercise, but one which eliminates lower-back strain, since your non-exercising arm is used to support the entire upper body, sheltering it from excess strain. Pull the dumbbell up into the midsection, and lower until the arm is extended all the way down, and then try a little harder to lower it even more. Maximize the stretch.

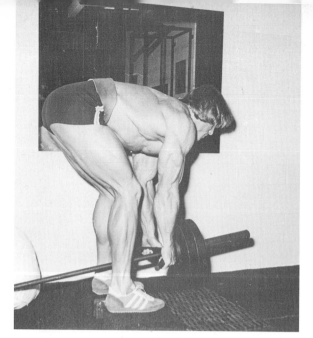

Champion bodybuilder Steve Davis likes T-bar rowing.

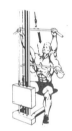

Lat Machine Pulldowns

This exercise has to be performed on a lat machine. Take a wide overgrip on the bar, and pull down as far as you can. This exercise is not as effective as the wide-grip chinning exercise, but does have the advantage that you can use less resistance and can therefore pull the bar lower and work your lats over a greater range of movement. You may pull to the front or the back of the neck.

John Cardillo demonstrates a great back exercise: bench rowing.

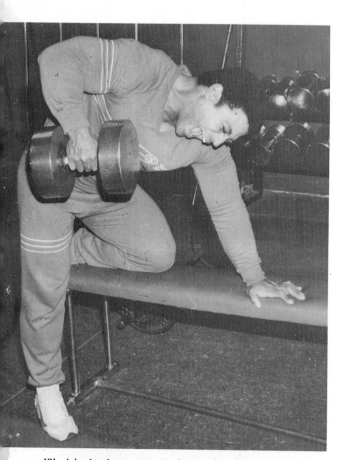

World physique star Mohamed Makkawy demonstrates a favorite back exercise, the single-arm dumbbell row.

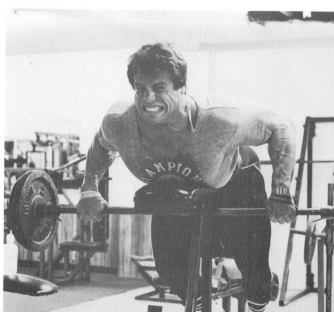

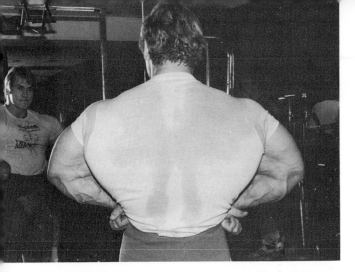

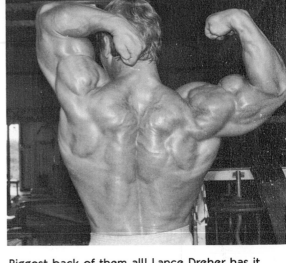

Massive is the only word for Lance Dreher's back.

Biggest back of them all! Lance Dreher has it.

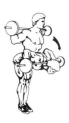

Good-Morning Exercise

Stand with legs set comfortably, a loaded barbell across your shoulders. Keeping your back flat, bend forward at the waist and straighten up. Hold your head as high as you can throughout the movement.

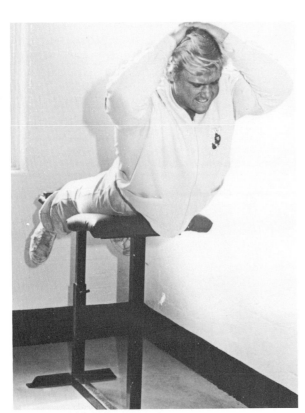

A must for the lower back: the prone hyperextension.

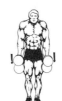

Barbell Shrug

Hold a barbell with a shoulder-width hand spacing while standing upright. The bar may be held in front of the body or behind it, as you prefer, and you may also substitute dumbbells for the barbell. Keeping the arms locked, raise the shoulders upwards towards the ears, as high as possible. Then rotate them backwards and down. Do not bend the knees. Concentrate on the up-down rotation of your shoulders. Some bodybuilders use a Universal bench press machine instead of free weights for this exercise. The Shrug is considered to be the best all-round trapezius-building movement.

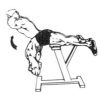

Prone Hyperextension

This is performed on an exercise unit especially designed for the job. Until recently, it was performed from a high bench or table. Place the legs and hips front downward on a suitable table top. A training partn[er] should hold your legs down to prevent your f[all]ing off the end. The upper body should be fr[ee to] rise up and down. Place your hands behind [your] head and lower your trunk towards the [floor.] Rise until your body is in a straight line. [...] and repeat.

In time, as your lumbar region str[ength] you may hold a barbell behind your h[ead as in] the Good-Morning exercise. This mo[vement is a] great favorite of Mike Mentzer's and [...] and both consider it one of the be[st] movements around.

20
SIZE IN THE THIGHS
Maxing Out the Upper Legs

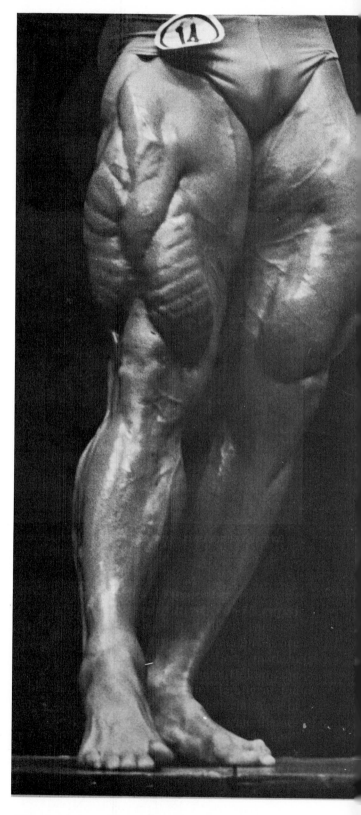

The phenomenal legs of Mr. Sensational—Tom Platz.

Thigh training has advanced greatly in the last few years. Twenty years ago, working the upper legs was accomplished with a few sets of regular squats—and that was it! With the advent of new machines and techniques, the competitive bodybuilders of today show entirely different thighs to those we knew in the 60's or before. In those days, cross-striations were unheard of. Only Vince Gironda had the upper _ard of. Only Vince Gironda had the upper _ separation and detail that is so important _ning today's contests. It would be true to _ver, that then, as now, the regular back _ing.

_squat is definitely _the_ growth ex- _impressiveness cannot be built _ept perhaps by the most ge- _n. If you are looking for _u must base your work- _ck squat. The other _nportant, are more _has its use, but _rovides, they

_ercise, but it _ht men until the _rior to that, lifters

would shoulder the weight after first standing it on end, and then they shuffled it into position on their shoulders.

One of the first to advocate training with the barbell squat was the Milo course, published at the beginning of this century. At that time, heavy weights were not recommended. Alan Calvert, who wrote the course, recommended a double-progression system, which even today cannot be bettered for beginning bodybuilders. It recommended twice as many repetitions for legs as for other parts. (Tom Platz would probably agree with this!) This is the way the Milo system worked:

You took a set poundage (on the light side) for an exercise (say the curl) and you proceeded to curl it five reps. You worked out every other day. On the second exercise day, you also did the movement five times. Then on the third exercise day, you increased the reps to six. After two more workout days you went on to seven, and so on, up to ten repetitions. When you had done ten reps twice with the starting weight, you increased the weight of the bar by five pounds, and began all over with five reps. In doing leg exercises, you started with ten reps and increased by two reps every third exercise day until you reached twenty. Then you increased the weight by ten pounds and dropped back to ten reps.

This system has several marked virtues. The first is that the body gets used to small amounts of progression, which definitely helps to avoid sticking points. In order to handle more and more and more weight, many of today's aspiring bodybuilders pile on the discs in order to maximize intensity and strength, only to find that they are quickly driving themselves into a musclebuilding stalemate.

The other virtue of the Milo system was that it was cyclic in nature. When you reached the maximum number of repetitions, it was a tremendous relief to increase the weight by only five pounds (or ten in the case of squats) and then go back to half the number of repetitions. It provided a sort of rest period (cycle training) in the first part of each series of progression. Even today, this system is great for the first five or six months of any newcomer's weight training. After that, it simply doesn't work.

Today, the greatest proponent of the regular back squat is Mr. Thomas Platz, who, it just

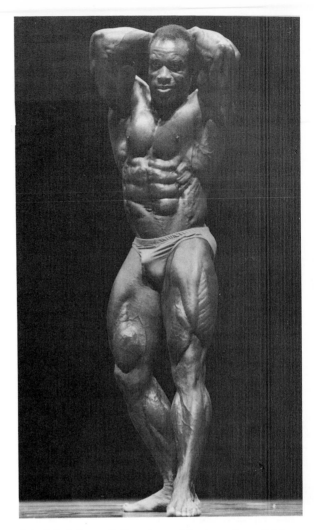

Britain's Johnny Fuller shows his ripped-up thighs.

happens, has the most phenomenal thigh development on Earth! Tom has some very specific advice on how to perform the squat properly. Most bodybuilders, Tom thinks, do not squat correctly. "I watch guys squat, and 80 percent of the time they don't do the movement right. Their feet are too far apart, their squat depth is too shallow, or they lean too far forward as they squat." Needless to say, when you lean too far forward, you put more stress on your buttocks than on your thighs. Let's drop in on the magnificent Platz as he prepares to squat.

The initial thing he does is some stretching. The hurdler's stretch for the front and back of the legs is first, and after that he does a hamstring stretch from a flat bench, keeping his legs locked tight.

What strikes you immediately when you observe Platz at leg-training time is that he is totally prepared for the job. He's wearing tight sweat pants, a regular leather lifting belt, plus a tight-fitting garment around his torso, "to enhance the secure feeling that you must have to squat properly and successfully." His shoes are weight-lifting boots with a raised heel. Platz doesn't recommend flat-footed squats in bare feet or tennis shoes.

He approaches the bar with a zeroed-in attitude. He means business. The bar taken from the racks is on his shoulders. A couple of steps back, and his feet are set—never wider than shoulder width, and usually considerably closer. His toes are pointed slightly outwards.

As Platz lowers into the squat, you know he is in total control. You feel it in your bones. The master is at work. His head is held high, his hands are placed on the bar about half way between his shoulders and the plates. The torso is flat-backed and upright. He lowers to parallel and beyond, and returns to the upright position. Even other professional bodybuilders stop what they are doing to watch Platz squat.

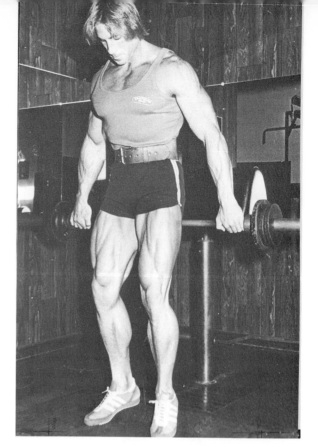

Steve Davis shows his form in the hack squat.

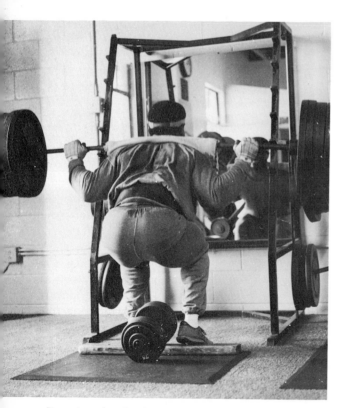

Bronston Austin, Jr., performs some heavy squats.

As he slowly sinks all the way down again, his knees travel out directly over his toes. He stays tight, keeping his back and torso muscles tensed, and . . . up again! The breathing is heavy. He breathes in before descending and squats on full lungs. Out jets the air as he straightens up. After the set, his jellyfish thighs make him yearn to sit down, but he resists the temptation. He walks around, paying back his temporary oxygen debt. The walking keeps the blood circulating, which helps him to recuperate quickly for the next set. To sit down would be encouraging workout lethargy. He may allow himself that luxury after completing his *entire* leg program.

Incidentally, Tom Platz had 20-inch thighs when he took up weight training. Now, at under 200 pounds of bodyweight, he has squatted with 600 pounds. He has also done an incredible 28 reps with 405 pounds, and 52 reps with 350. And according to observer Bill Reynolds, prior to 1977, Platz was doing ten straight minutes of squatting with 225 pounds!! Platz's *Leg Training Manual* is absolute "must" reading for all dedicated bodybuilders.

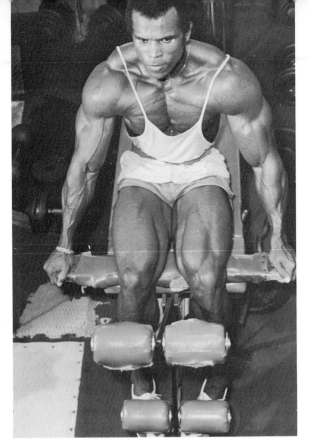

Thigh extensions done Nubret-style.

The usefulness of the thigh extension is limited to its muscle-isolating effect. The quads are actually separated during the movement, which may contribute to improved appearance on contest day when you have dieted off all the fat. Needless to say, the thigh extensions themselves will not remove fat.

Another negative aspect of thigh extensions is that they should not be performed at a time when you are trying to build up squat power. They would lessen your gains in squatting poundage.

Mohamed Makkawy, the Egyptian Grand Prix champion, uses the thigh extension in a unique way. He does his thigh extensions lying down with his back flat on the bench. That carries the muscle-isolating effect into the upper part of the thighs, near the groin. This little-known method improved the separation of Mohamed's entire thigh area 100 percent.

Not to be neglected are the thigh biceps. You should exercise them during every leg workout. If you vary the angle at which you perform leg curls, you will hit different parts of the leg biceps, and accordingly maximize the development in those areas.

Yes, the king of exercises, the squat, will help your overall gains along more than any other movement. You should beware, however, of doing too much. An excessive number of sets with maximum weights can lead to overtraining. It is seldom advisable to squat more than twice a week, and even then, one session should be somewhat watered down. In other words, don't shoot for two weekly squat workouts using the training-to-failure technique.

After squatting, you should (unless you are a beginner) employ at least one other frontal thigh exercise. The hack squat is a good supplementary movement. Added size and shape can result from hacks.

The thigh extension exercise is useless, at least as a thigh *builder*. It is a very popular movement, however, and used by bodybuilders at all stages. Its charm may be that it is a delight to behold! There you are, your thighs held in place by a bench, your lower legs pumping up and down. It looks like something is working. But where's the size? The truth of the matter is that the thigh extension is a fantastic *knee* exercise, and that's it!

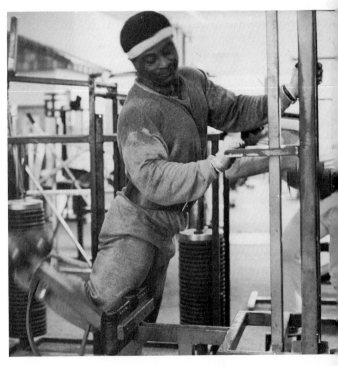

Mr. America contender Bronston Austin, Jr., works on the single-leg thigh curl at Gold's Gym.

113

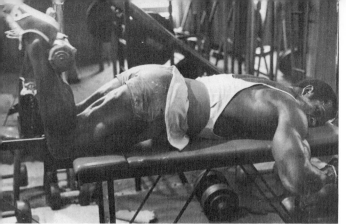
Serge Nubret performs the thigh curl.

When training the thighs, pay attention to developing proportion. For instance, if you have just done heavy quarter squats for the thighs, you want to guard against developing "turnip thighs" (large upper thighs, small lower thighs). In order to balance development, you should now work the lower thigh with some specialized movements, such as the sissy squat, or hack lift.

Vince Gironda knows a lot about thigh balance and development. In fact, he was giving thought to the various thigh muscles and their relationship to one another thirty years ago, when the bodybuilders who won Mr. Universe contests had turnip thighs.

Gironda has voiced his disaffection for the regular back squat by saying, "They build butts, not thighs." It is known that he does not have squat stands in his North Hollywood gym. But what his critics fail to acknowledge is that Gironda does recommend certain types of squats. Usually, his gym members are directed towards the Smith machine. Because of its fixed, vertical-slide position, the Smith machine enables the exerciser to place his feet farther forward than he could in a free-weight squat with a barbell. Therefore more stress is thrown on the entire thigh area, rather than the hips and butt.

The question is often asked, "Is the leg press as effective an exercise as the regular back squat?" The questioner expects the answer to be *yes*, since the leg press appears at first glance to involve a squatting-type leg movement. More than likely, the questioner does not like the regular squat. He either hasn't the wind for it, or it makes him feel like throwing up, or it is just too close to downright hard work.

Great weights can be hoisted using the leg press, and the apparatus is useful in working the thigh relatively comfortably from a variety of an-gles (you can alter foot placing dramatically). But as an overall-thigh exercise, the leg press is definitely inferior to the squat, which is truly the most effective thigh builder currently known to mankind. Not the answer you were looking for? Maybe not, but it's the truth! *Here are the best leg exercises.*

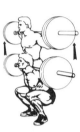

The Squat
Entire Thigh Area (6–20 reps per set)
Take a weight from a pair of squat racks and hold it, hands on bar, at the back of your neck. If needed, place your heels on a two-by-four block of wood to improve balance. Some people just cannot squat flat-footed. It forces them to adopt a very wide foot stance, and even so, they are forced to lean too far forwards when squatting down.

Breathe in deeply before squatting down. Keep your back flat and your head up throughout the movement. Breathe out forcefully as you raise up.

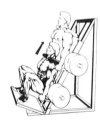

The Hack Squat
Mid and Lower Thigh (10–15 reps each set)
Position yourself on a hack machine. Lower and raise yourself by bending and straightening your legs. Depending on the set-up of machine you use, you may find it advantageous to perform the hack machine exercise with your feet placed in varying positions. (Heels together with toes pointing outwards will develop the lateral section of the thigh.) Also, you may want to experiment by keeping your knees together, or alternatively, you may want to hold them out to the sides.

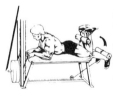

Leg Curls
Thigh biceps (12–15 reps each set)
Lie on a thigh curl machine, face down. Hook your heels under the lift bar and proceed to curl your legs upwards in unison. Concentrate on securing the "feel" in the backs of your legs. Do not bounce the weight up after the legs straighten, but rather pause and start the curl slowly and deliberately.

Thigh Extensions
Lower and Middle Thigh
(10–15 reps each set)

Sit on a thigh-extension machine with the tops of your feet (at the ankle flexion point) affixed under the lift pad. Start raising the weight by extending both legs together. Do not "kick" the weight up. Start the lift slowly. If the machine you are using starts to race, you are exerting too much explosive force. Slow down and make the muscles "feel it."

The Leg Press

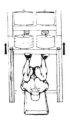

This is almost like an inverted squat. Many bodybuilders prefer the leg press because it allows full concentration on the leg action without great involvement of the hip area. It is generally accepted, with good reason, that the leg press is *not* as effective a leg builder as the back squat, but it is certainly easier on the lungs.

Place your feet about 1 foot (30 cm) apart under the plate of the apparatus, and press upwards until the legs straighten. Lower, and repeat. If you get stuck, aid the legs by using your hands to press on the thighs.

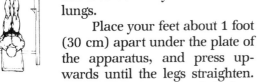

Massive legs are important for contest winning.

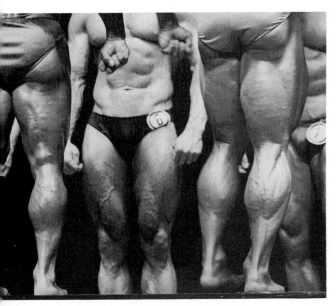

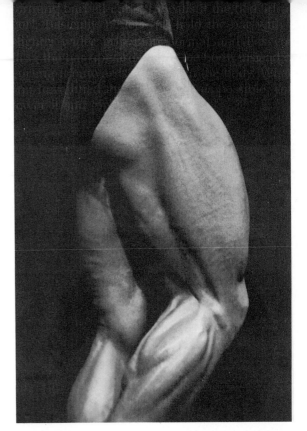

Leg development must be complete from all angles.

Sissy Squat

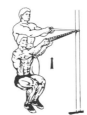

This is a very specialized movement, designed principally to work the lower thigh area. Because of the unusual angle at which the exercise is performed, this movement is done with either no weight or only a moderate poundage. (Weight can be added either by holding a barbell in front of the shoulders or by holding dumbbells at arm's length at the sides.) The name "sissy squat" is not intended to denote that the exercise is easy, or for sissies. Quite the contrary. The name is derived from a character in Greek mythology, Sisyphus, whose eternal punishment by the gods consisted of having to roll a huge rock up a mountainside, only to have it roll down, over and over again.

The exercise is a little tricky. Adopt a position with your feet about 18 inches (45 cm) apart. Rise up on your toes, and lower into a squat while leaning as far back as possible. The point to bear in mind is to keep your thigh and torso in the same plane throughout the exercise. If performance is difficult, then hold onto the back of a chair to prevent loss of balance.

21
CALVES
Building the Lower Legs

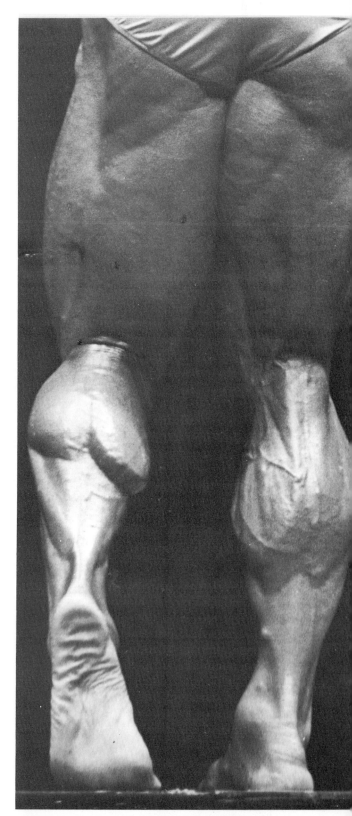

Incredible is the only word for Tom Platz's lower legs.

Calves used to be the bugbear of bodybuilders all over the world. Hardly anyone apart from Grimek had them in the old days. Then came the 50's, and even then, pretty few had them. Reeves and Delinger had great calf development, of course, but it wasn't until the introduction and nationwide use of the standing calf machine enabled bodybuilders to use very heavy poundages each leg workout that the lower legs really started to blossom. Today we also have the seated calf machine and the leg press apparatus to help keep the calves growing, so it is no longer considered "impossible" to develop the calf muscle to any great degree.

Of course, if an individual doesn't have a sufficient number of muscle cells (genetic potential), he will certainly find it impossible to develop Mike Mentzer calves.

Many black men have a "high" calf, which in extreme cases means that they will not be able to build a balanced or big lower leg. Ironically, and in seeming contradiction to the above, some of the best calves in the business belong to black men. Witness the lower-leg development of Sergio Oliva, Johnny Fuller, Bertil Fox, and Chris Dickerson!

One of the first men to do a real job on his calves was the many-time Mr. Universe Reg Park. At the time of winning the Mr. Britain, Reg had underdeveloped lower legs. But he totally remodelled them by working them on a daily basis, with ever-increasing weight loads, on a standing calf machine. At times when he was unable to use the machine, Reg would perform donkey calf raises with two heavy training partners sitting across his back. Just before the Mr. Universe contest, which he won, Park was training his calves twice a day. Park ultimately put four inches on his calves with this heavy progressive-resistance training. How heavy? He used up to 800 pounds of resistance on the standing calf raise.

Reg Park was the early hero of another physique star: none other than Arnold Schwarzenegger, the Austrian Oak. Curiously, Arnold also had difficulty in developing his lower legs. He decided to use Park's method of working the calf every day with extremely heavy weights. It worked so well, talk went around that Arnold had actually had silicone implants—a rumor with absolutely no foundation.

Way back in the last century when men wore tights, it was common practice for men to wear false calves, just as today we have jackets fitted with shoulder pads to give the visual appearance of added width. Eugen Sandow, known as the father of modern bodybuilding, actually did wear false calves—until he developed a fine set of his own after a couple of years of training.

Another bodybuilder who has really fine underpinnings is Boyer Coe. I watched carefully as he exercised them. Amazingly, Boyer spends at least twenty minutes each workout *stretching* his calves. He does this by standing on a high block without any weights, stretching up as high as he can, and then lowering down to maximize the effect. At this stage, Boyer is only interested in getting a full and complete stretching action. Later on in the workout Boyer trains his lower legs with resistance exercise (calf machines) and follows the traditional pattern of working them with about 5 sets of 15–20 reps.

Vince Gironda, another believer in maximum flexibility, is adamantly opposed to doing calf exercises barefooted. He says, "It is best to do your calf work on a 6-inch block covered with a ½-inch layer of rubber padding."

Larry Scott, a pupil of Gironda's, goes one step further. He follows Vince's advice to the letter but adds a new twist. "I prefer donkey calf raises, but when the calves start to burn really painfully, I bend my knees slightly to allow the pump to leave my lower legs and circulate more easily. This takes the pain away and allows me to continue on with blitzing my lower legs."

Way back in the late 40's and early 50's, the bodybuilding world was in a state of shock over the superb calf development of Steve Reeves. No one could figure out how he got such shapely and well-developed lower legs. Writers and physical culture experts concluded that Reeves had largely built his calves as a paper boy, cycling up and down the hills of Oakland, California. This was quoted as gospel truth for a decade, but was discounted when Reeves exclaimed in an interview published in *MuscleMag International*: "There were no hills on my paper route!"

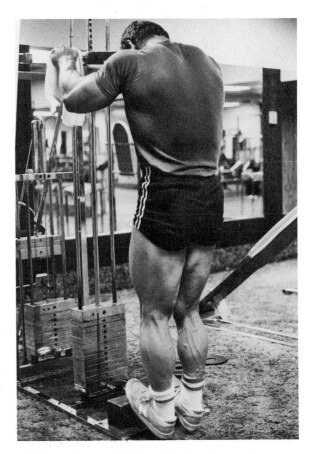

Lance Dreher works his calves hard every leg — training day.

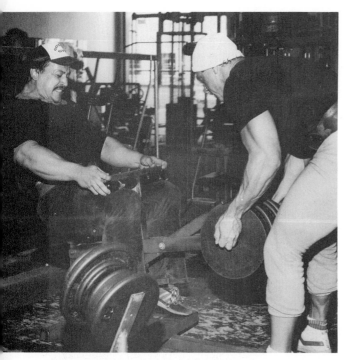

Casey Viator gives everything to a set of seated calf exercises. Note how his training partner aids with the last few reps.

In actual fact, Reeves worked his calves with a heel-raise machine and with donkey calf raises. He also *redesigned* his walk. Yes, his walk! He would rise up and down on his toes as he walked, so that his calves were put through an almost full range of extensions whenever he walked anywhere. His dynamic walking style can still be seen in some of his *Hercules* movies, and it became a trademark of his virility and healthy, lust-for-life appearance. Ultimately, Reeves took his walk even further and developed a longer stride and a more pronounced arm swing. This became known as the "power walk," and a book by Reeves under the same title was recently published in the USA. Needless to say, Reeves only uses the power walking style when exercising. You will hardly catch him walking down Wilshire Boulevard using such exaggerated walking style.

The point is often raised that those with high calves should not be penalized in a contest. "After all," the argument goes, "many black men, and not a few white ones, do not have the potential for building calves. Should they lose a contest just because they have been given a particular structure by Mother Nature?"

The answer, of course, is, "Too bad!" Nature may have given us poor calf genetics, poor arm shape, poor leg development, lousy-looking abs. So what! A contest has to go to the best-developed, best-proportioned guy. The fact that he has been dealt a bum hand as far as genetics is concerned is no reason to hand him an award. A 5 foot 6 man won't make a national basketball team, and a man with 20-inch arms going steady with 14-inch underpins will not win a Mr. Olympia. Nor should he, whatever his inherited genetics.

Who has the best calf development of all time? In spite of the fact that many champions have remarkable lower leg development, I think that for all round shape, definition and size, the "World's Greatest-looking Calf" title should go to the one and only Chris Dickerson.

Going all out in his calf training: Roy Callendar, who is now running a successful gym in Barbados.

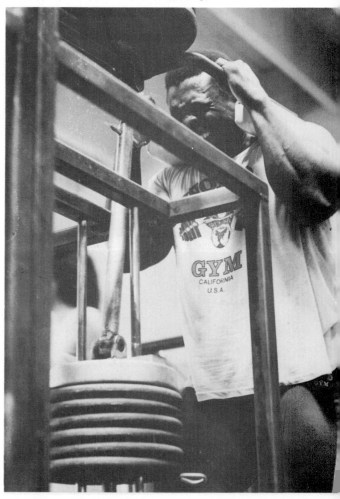

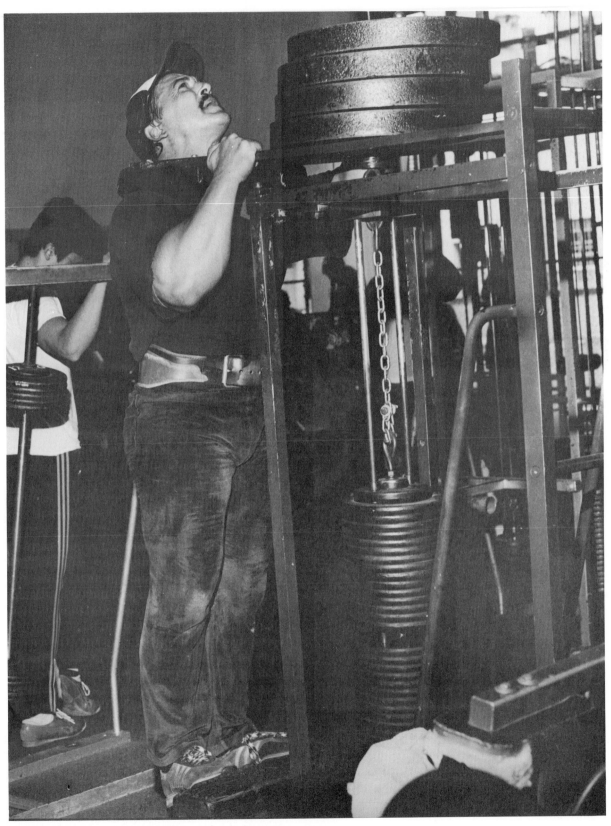

Standing calf raise as performed by superstar Casey Viator.

Donkey Calf Raise

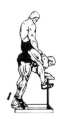

There is no doubt that the bent-over position one adopts for the donkey calf raise exercise does something very special for the lower legs. This exercise is a great favorite of Mr. Olympia Frank Zane. Lean on a bench or table top so that your upper body is comfortably supported parallel to the floor. Have a training partner sit on your lower back, over the hip area. Rise up and down on your toes until you cannot perform another rep. Use a 4-inch block under your toes to give greater range to the foot movement. You should always aim to perform at least 20 reps in this exercise.

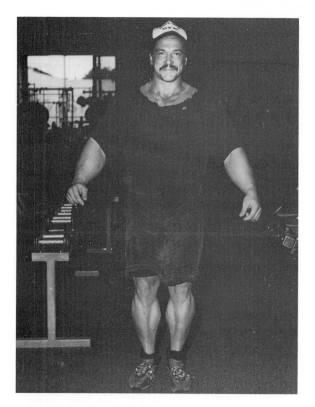

Casey Viator shows off his super-sized calf development.

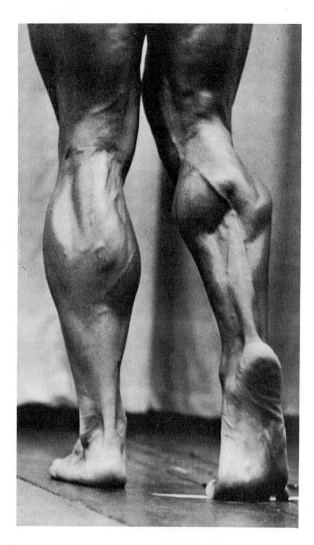

The super calves of Mike Mentzer.

Standing Calf Raise

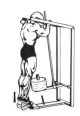

It is important that the calf machine you use is capable of loading on heavy weights. The apparatus should either carry a huge stack of weights or else be set up with a leverage benefit, so that comparatively small weights give a considerably increased overall load.

Rise up and down on your toes without excessive knee bending and without bouncing at the bottom of the movement.

Seated Calf Raise

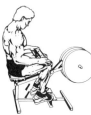

This exercise, too, is performed on a special leverage machine. The principal muscle worked in this movement is the ,*soleus* rather than the *gastrocnemius*. Perform as many heel raises as you can, concentrating on maximizing total calf stretch with each repetition.

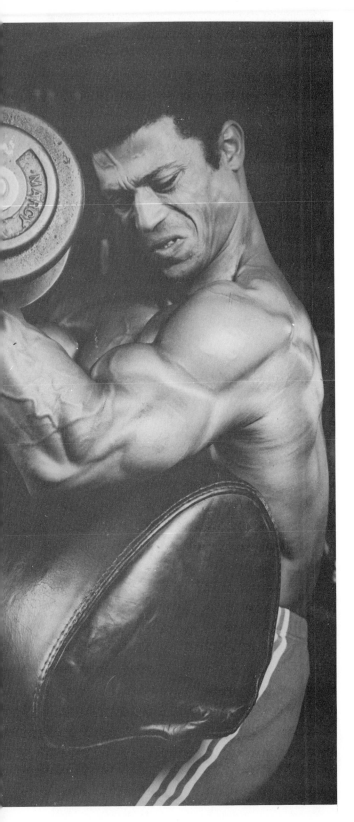

Egypt's Mohamed Makkawy performs Scott curls.

22
ARMS
Filling Out Your Sleeves— But Quick

Let's clear the air on one aspect of arm training: it *may* be possible to build large arms with three sets of biceps and three sets of triceps exercises, but it hasn't often been done. In thirty years I have only known one case where a pair of large arms were developed on such a limited schedule, but those arms were "naturally" large to begin with!

To build arms, really *build* them, you need to work on a regular basis using about 10–15 sets for biceps and 10–15 sets for triceps—minimum! Some experts may disagree with this. So be it. I have no axe to grind. My recommendations are based solely on observation and experience.

Perhaps one day there will be a concentrated training method that can activate the deepest muscle fibres of the arms with just *one* set of exercises. Ultimately, technology may allow us to "hit them" completely with a few seconds of exhausting stimulation, but until someone invents it, be prepared to perform plenty of quality sets and reps.

When you compare the bodybuilders of the 40's and 50's with the champions of today, you

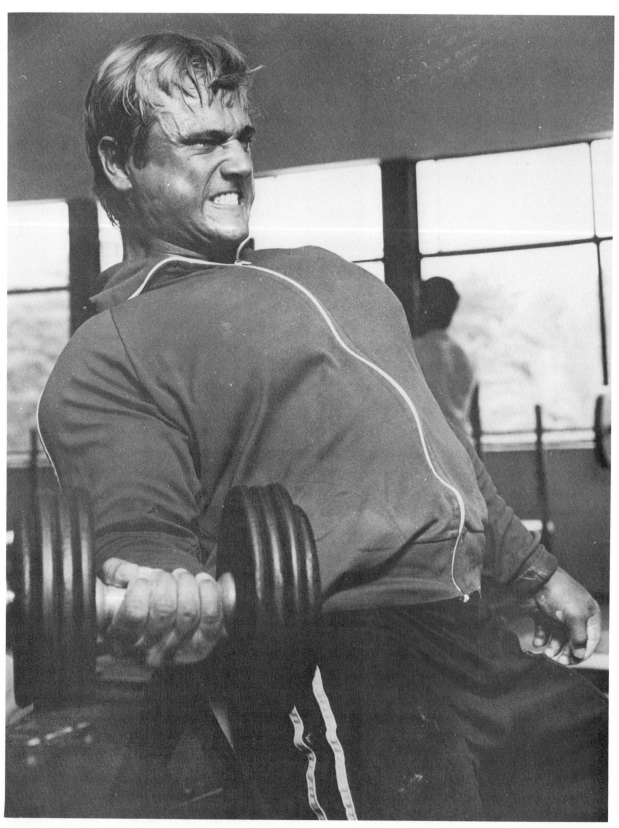

One arm curls as performed by Tom Platz.

can see that arm development has advanced more than the development of other body parts.

We have come a long way from the Greek ideal by which the neck, calf, and flexed upper arm were considered to be in perfect harmony if they measured the same. Until the middle of this century most top bodybuilders aimed for this ideal and more or less achieved it. Steve Reeves achieved a calf, upper arm, and neck development of 18 inches; so did John Grimek, Clancy Ross, Roy Hilligen, Armand Tanny, Reg Park, and scores of others.

Today, we have title winners with 17-inch calves and necks but 20-inch arms. Some have an even greater differential. The purists—and perhaps in my heart of hearts I am one, too—greatly disparage this new trend. "It is wrong," they say. "No man should have upper arms that much bigger than his calves." Right or wrong, the trend is with us. It is in vogue to have huge upper arms, and many bodybuilders feel: the bigger the better.

It is a good idea to work the upper arms with at least one heavy exercise and one or two lighter, pumping movements.

For the biceps, the best heavy or "quality" movements are:

1. Barbell curl
2. Incline dumbbell curl
3. Seated dumbbell curl

For the triceps, the best heavy or "quality" movements are:

1. Close-grip EZ curl bar bench press
2. Parallel bar dips
3. Lying triceps barbell stretch

It is recommended that you begin your biceps and triceps routines with one of these quality exercises.

Let me give you some idea of how some of the big-armed men of muscledom start their biceps routines. Robby Robinson, Mike Mentzer, Roy Callender, Arnold Schwarzenegger, Franco Columbu, Ed Corney, Dave Draper, Rick Wayne, all begin with the basic barbell curl. Guys like Kal Szkalak, Samir Bannout, Greg DeFerro, Tom Platz, Mike Katz, Danny Padilla begin with seated or incline dumbbell curls.

Remember what I said: quality first.

When it comes to triceps, there are literally hundreds of movements for this area. Serge Nubret, who has outstanding arms, begins his routine with the lying triceps stretch, and so do Danny Padilla, Kal Szkalak, and Lou Ferrigno. Larry Scott, who for years had the world's big-

A determined effort by bodybuilding great Greg DeFerro.

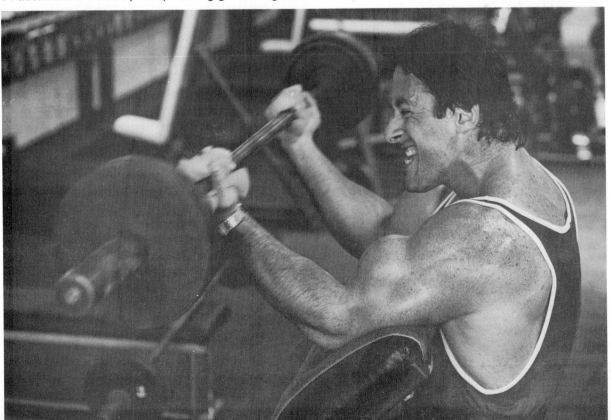

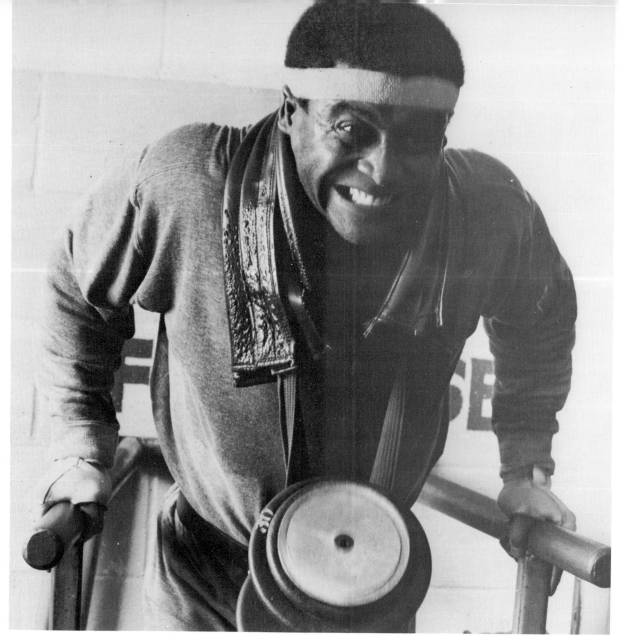

Bronston Austin, Jr., performs dips with weight for triceps.

gest arms, begins his triceps workout with the narrow-grip EZ curl bar bench press, as do Tom Platz, Frank Zane, and Arnold Schwarzenegger. Again, quality first.

There is one triceps exercise that virtually everybody uses in his routine: No doubt it is such a favorite because it seems like such a "pure" exercise. Right now I cannot think of a single champion who does not use it regularly. The stress is pretty even throughout the movement, and no appreciable balance is needed to perform a set. Although this isolation exercise is popular and gets you a good pump, it is not a size builder in the sense of a combination or "natural" exercise such as the close-grip bench press or the parallel bar dip. As one expert said, "You want big triceps? Go for parallel bar dips. When you can do 20 reps with a 100-pound dumbbell hanging from your waist, you'll have 'em."

After you have been weight training for a while, you will find (when you think about it) that certain arm exercises seem to be giving results, while others just don't. If you think nothing much is happening, then your observations are probably correct.

Especially avoid any exercise that gives you pain or discomfort in the elbow region. There are several triceps movements which can contribute to *tendinitis* (inflammation of the tendon) in the elbow. You must immediately stop using such an exercise or else cut down drastically on the weight you were using. Let's assume you have worked up to using 6 reps with 120 pounds in the lat-machine pressdowns exercise, but the pain is unbearable. Either stop the exercise entirely or push it to the end of your arm routine and merely perform a few pumping sets of 20 reps with a far lighter weight!

Apart from proportion, there are four vital qualities that make up a great arm:
1. You need *size*. This includes thickness and roundness from the top of the arm near the shoulder to the bottom near the elbow.
2. You need good *shape*. This is largely hereditary. Ideal examples of shapely biceps are Arnold Schwarzenegger, Larry Scott, and Robby Robinson. Men known for their triceps include Frank Zane, Dennis Tinerino, and Mohamed Makkawy.
3. You need *separation*, the distinct delineation of the various muscles that make up an arm.
4. You need *vascularity* and *definition*. The skin must be "thin" with a low fat percentage. Veins grow in size along with the arms, especially if plenty of pump is achieved in your workouts.

I mentioned earlier how some top bodybuilders start their arm training, and that was true; but remember that many bodybuilders change their routines around. A bodybuilder who usually starts his arm routine with barbell curls may suddenly switch to starting with chins, or even concentration curls. This is what bodybuilding is all about: shocking the muscles into growth. Lou Ferrigno, for example, changes his arm exercises every month, and even from workout to workout he may change the angles if he feels the urge. He might, for example, do incline curls on a 45-degree bench one day but set it at a 30-degree angle the next day. Alternatively, he may curl the dumbbells out a little farther from the body than usual.

You, too, may want to alter your arm training angles from time to time. You can, for example, try dumbbell curling with palms facing upwards one day, and the next day do it with your palms facing inwards.

Can you change the shape of your arms? Yes and no. Confusing? Well, you can add shape to your triceps by working, say, the outer triceps section very hard. This will give an attractive appearance to the arm, especially when it is in the straight or "hang" position. Alternatively, you can add impressiveness through exercises that work the lower triceps near the elbow.

The biceps are a little more stubborn. For example, by working the lower biceps on a shallow-angle Scott bench, you will "lengthen" the biceps only slightly; and by training hard on concentration peak-contraction curls, you will slightly increase the height of your biceps. In short, you cannot significantly change your inherited arm shape.

Triceps pushdowns. Reid Schindle likes to use a rope to maximize the effect.

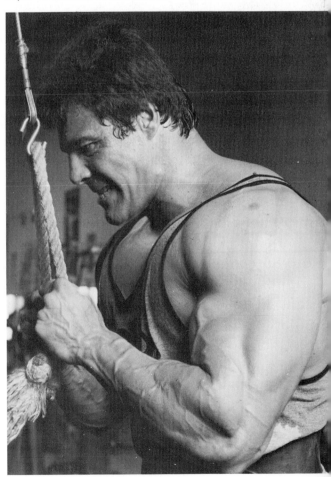

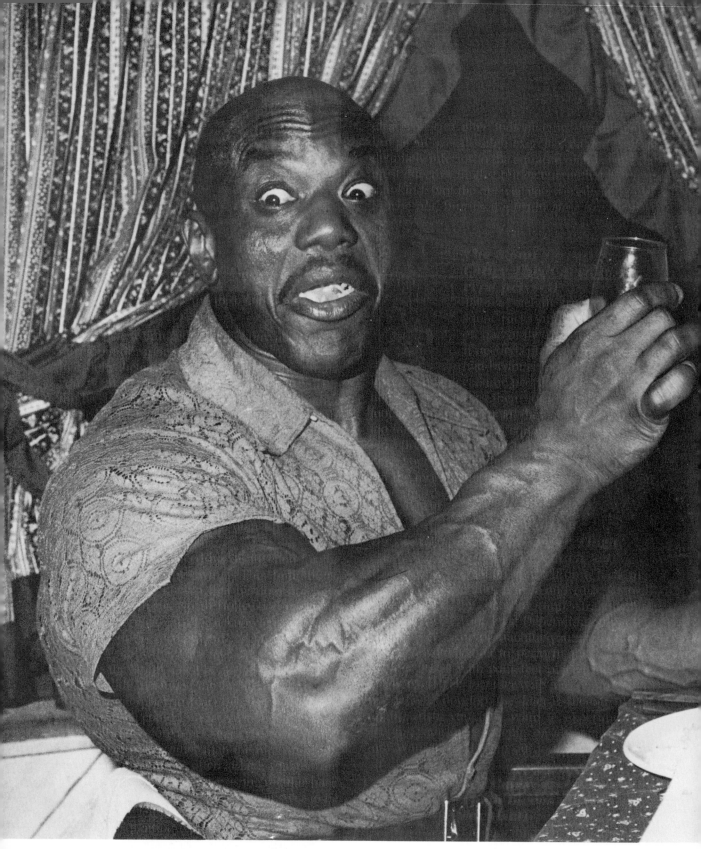

The great Sergio jokes around while partaking of a little wine.

Biceps Exercises

The Incline Dumbbell Curl

Lie back on an incline bench slanted at about 45 degrees. Hold two dumbbells in the arms-down position. It does not matter whether you start the movement with your palms facing inwards or upwards. The only difference is that the forearms are brought more into play when the palms are facing inwards.

Keep your head back on the bench and curl up both dumbbells simultaneously. Your seat should not come up from the bench at any time during the curl, since that would aid the biceps in getting the weight up and therefore relieve them of some of their work. If they do less work, how can they build up size or strength?

As soon as the dumbbells reach shoulder level, lower, and repeat. Some bodybuilders actually tense their biceps at the end of the curl when the dumbbells are at shoulder level. This is just another way of maximizing intensity, and it is up to you whether you choose to do it.

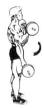

Barbell Curl

Generally considered the king of biceps builders, the regular barbell curl has contributed to more 20-inch arms than any other movement. Hold the bar slightly wider than shoulder width, and keep your elbows close to your body as you curl the weight upwards until it is under your chin.

There are two distinct styles of doing this exercise: *strictly* (no leaning back during the movement, starting from a straight-arm position, using absolutely no body motion or "swing"), or *cheating* (hoisting the weight up by turning the trunk of your body into a pendulum on which the barbell can rely for added momentum). Both methods are workable, and most successful bodybuilders get best results by doing at least the first 6 or 8 repetitions in strict style and then finishing off the harder last 3 or 4 repetitions with a cheating motion.

Vince Gironda has his own way of per- forming barbell curls. He calls it the body-drag curl. Basically, he lets you hold the bar with a slightly wider grip than normal and has you drag the bar upwards along the body, instead of curling it outwards away from the body. When you have lifted the bar as high as possible, you lower it and repeat.

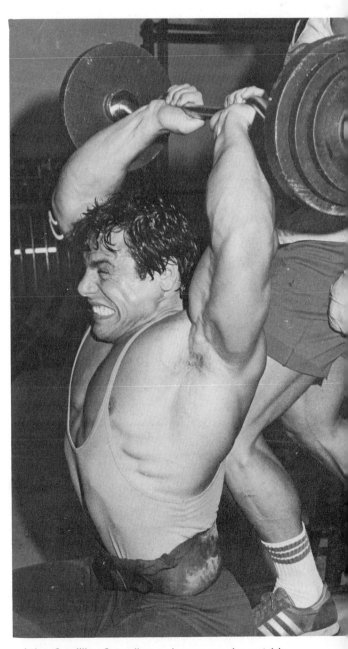

John Cardillo, Canadian colossus, works out his triceps with an "easy curl" bar.

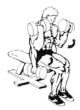

Alternate Dumbbell Curl

This exercise is a great favorite of champion bodybuilder Rocky DeFerro. It works the biceps more directly than the two-handed dumbbell curl, since it prevents undue leanback or cheating.

Perform the movement by sitting erect and first curling one dumbbell. Then, as you lower it, curl the other arm. Lower slowly, and do not swing the bells up with any added body motion.

Concentration Curl

Sit at the end of a bench. Exercise only one arm at a time, resting your elbow on the inside of the thigh (above the knee). Rest the non-exercising hand on your free leg. Slowly curl the straight arm upwards, then lower it at the same speed. Concentrate intently on the biceps muscle as it contracts each time the dumbbell is curled upwards. Immediately after training one arm, do an identical number of repetitions with the other arm.

Arnold Schwarzenegger has another version of this curl, one he feels has contributed more to his monumental biceps size and peak than any other. He places one hand on a low

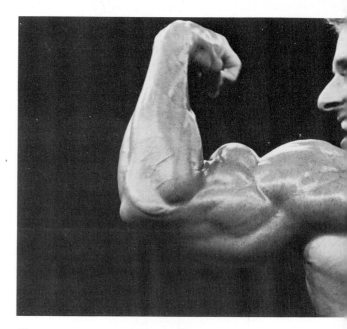

The massive arm of Greg DeFerro.

stool or exercise bench and holds a dumbbell at arm's length hanging downwards. Arnold makes a point of keeping his shoulder low throughout this exercise. This movement does in fact "hit" the biceps in an unusual fashion. It may take you a few workouts to get the hang of it, but once you do, I am sure you will benefit enormously.

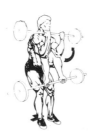

Scott Curls

Adopt a position with your arms over a preacher (Scott) bench. Hold either a barbell (as shown) or a pair of dumbbells. Curl up to the chin, then lower slowly. Do not bounce the weights when the arms are in the straight position. Raise and repeat.

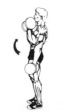

Standing Dumbbell Curl

Adopt a comfortable standing position with your feet about 18 inches (45 cm) apart. Holding dumbbells in both hands, curl both arms simultaneously until the dumbbells are next to your shoulders. Start with your palms facing inwards. As you raise the weights, turn your wrists so that the palms are facing upwards. Lower the bells slowly, and repeat.

Superstar Tom Platz shows his style in the barbell curl.

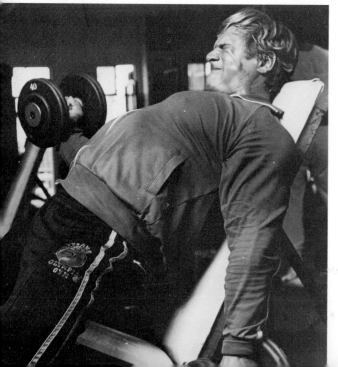

128

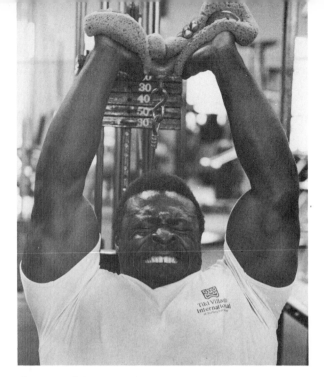

Super training: Roy Callendar working triceps.

Flat Bench Lying Dumbbell Curl

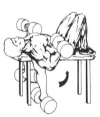

This is performed in the same way as the incline dumbbell curl, except that the bench is completely flat. Most people of average height or taller will need a comparatively high bench, so that the dumbbells don't hit the floor at the bottom of the curl.

Because of the unusual position, you may find that this exercise puts too much stress on your arms. It is therefore advisable to start this exercise with comparatively light weights.

Undergrip Close-Hand Chin

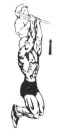

This is a terrific biceps building exercise with a difference. Instead of the arm moving from the body, your body gets curled towards the arm—rather like the proverbial tail wagging the dog.

Grasp an overhead horizontal bar with an undergrip so that your little fingers are 6–12 inches (15–30 cm) apart. Starting from a "dead hang" position with arms entirely straight, pull upwards until your chin is above the level of the bar. Lower under control, and repeat.

Triceps Exercises

Close-Grip Bench Press

This is a great favorite with Larry Scott, the first Mr. Olympia, who said it has given him more triceps development than any other. Lie face up on a flat bench, feet firmly planted on the floor. Take a fairly heavy barbell (EZ curl bars are the most popular among the pros) from the racks (or have a partner hand it to you). Use a narrow grip so your hands are only 2–3 inches (5–9 cm) apart. Keeping your elbows close to your body, lower the weight to your lower breastbone, and immediately push upwards. Larry Scott and Dennis Tinerino use more than 250 pounds for this movement, but if you are new to this or any other exercise, you should start by using only light weights.

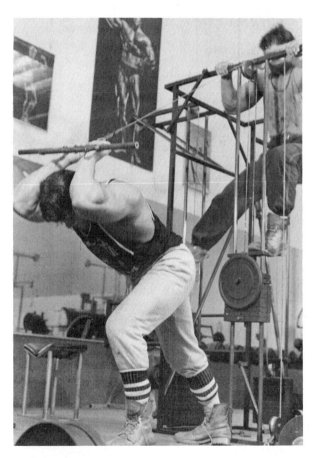

The Barbarians are coming! Peter Paul uses the additional weight of his brother David on the triceps machine.

129

Mr. America 1981, Tim Belknap, shows what it took to gain the title.

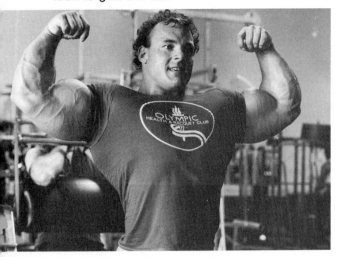

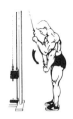

Pressdowns on Lat Machine

Was there ever a bodybuilder who didn't spend a great deal of time and effort performing this exercise? Start by holding a lat-machine bar with your hands 2–8 inches (5–20 cm) apart. Now press downwards until the arms are straight. Return, and repeat. Most bodybuilders keep their elbows at their sides during this movement. A few, such as Dennis Tinerino, deliberately hold the elbows out to the sides and "lean" into the exercise. The choice is yours.

Bertil Fox. His arms are among the best in the world.

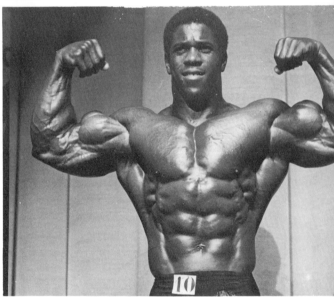

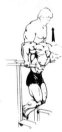

Parallel Bar Dips

Mike Mentzer endorses this exercise. Start with arms straight, feet tucked up under the torso. Lower (dip) while keeping elbows close to the body, then raise and return. As you get strong enough to perform 10–12 repetitions, add weight either by "holding" a dumbbell between the thighs while crossing your legs at the ankle, or by attaching iron discs to a "dipping belt" designed especially for the task.

The magic arm of Mr. Universe Lance Dreher.

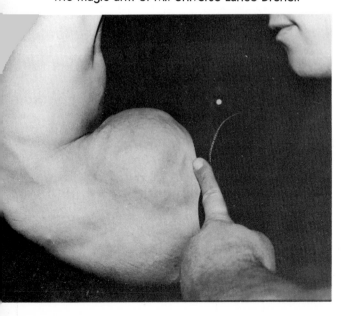

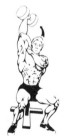

Single-Arm Dumbbell Triceps Stretch

Kal Szkalak favors this triceps exercise, which develops the lower triceps area expecially. With practice, it is possible to handle very heavy poundages— some top bodybuilders use dumbbells of 100 pounds or more—but it is not always advisable to use excessive weights in this particular movement, since they may put too much strain on your elbow joints and their surrounding ligaments. Beware of bouncing the weight out of the "low" part of the movement: this, too, can cause elbow problems.

Bent-Over Triceps Kickbacks

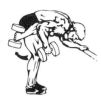

Another Larry Scott favorite. Bend over so that your torso is parallel to the floor. Hold a dumbbell in one hand and hold onto a rail with the other hand. Raise and lower the dumbbell at an even rate, keeping the upper arm in line with your torso and parallel to the floor. Keep your upper arm tight against your waist throughout.

Seated Triceps Dumbbell Extension

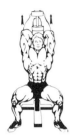

Hold a single dumbbell behind your back, with your upper arms as close to your ears as possible. Raise and lower the weight while keeping your upper arms vertical.

Lying Triceps Stretch

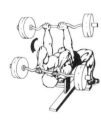

Lie on your back as shown, and hold an EZ curl bar at arm's length. Lower it slowly to the forehead, and raise again to arm's length. This exercise works the entire triceps area.

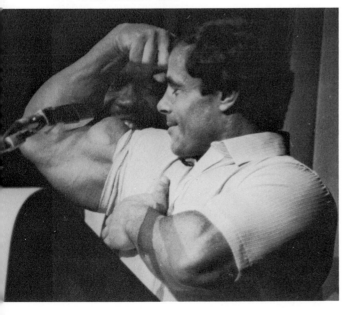

Franco is always popular with audiences. Here he shows his massive arm.

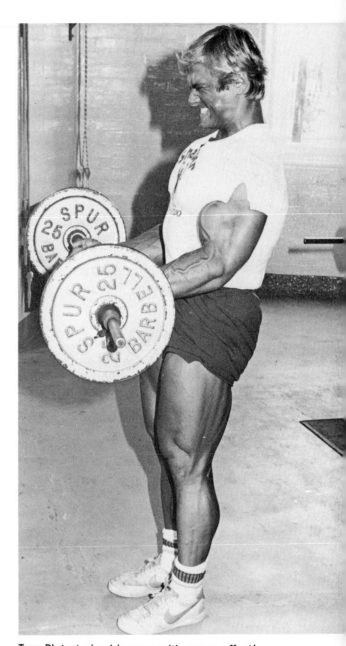

Tom Platz trains his arms with super effort!

Bent-over Lat-Machine Extensions

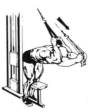

Assume a bent-over, strongly balanced position, holding a straight triceps bar attached to a lat-machine setup. Keeping the upper arms locked straight throughout the exercise, extend the forearms. Start the movement slowly without jerking. This is an excellent exercise for the outer head of the triceps.

23
FOREARMS
Bringing the Lower Arms Up

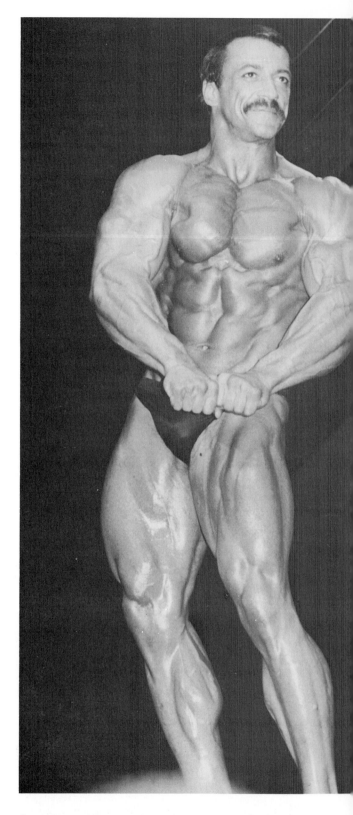

Long known for his super forearms—Casey Viator of Beverly Hills.

Until fairly recently top bodybuilders did no specific forearm exercises. Since every exercise (yes, even squats) works the lower arms in some way, it was argued that special forearm movements were not needed. Only Californian Chuck Sipes exercised his forearms individually with isolation movements. He was so different in his approach that even Arnold Schwarzenegger was heard to say, "Sipes spends too much time working with his forearms."

But times change, and now with the age of specialization upon us, most bodybuilders find time to train their forearms two or three times a week.

Casey Viator does. Casey, who is among the top three in the world with regard to forearms, openly admits that his forearms gave him trouble in the beginning of his bodybuilding career. "It's only been through hard and persistent training," he says "that I've been able to build up my forearms."

But not everybody trains their lower arms, nor do they need to. Michael Mentzer doesn't. Ironically, his forearms are unparallelled for quality and size. He attributes their growth to a combination of "lucky genetics" and the fact that his heavy duty style of training forces him to grip the dumbbells and barbells with extreme pressure and prolongs the forearm's involvement through a series of forced and even negative repetitions.

Many bodybuilders complain that as they complete a set, especially a high-repetition or heavy-duty set, their forearms "blow up" and fatigue earlier than the muscle they are supposed to be working. This can happen with exercises like chins, curls, and even upright rowing, and it's largely due to the individual's particular arrangement of muscle origins and insertions. Of course it is a source of annoyance to those who experience it, but those of us with puny, underdeveloped forearms would *love* them to blow up while we are doing sundry exercises, because our lower arms cannot be galvanized into significant development however we try!

Great forearms have belonged to only a handful of bodybuilders. Apart from Sipes, Viator, and Mentzer, men like Dave Draper,

Larry Scott, Tim Belknap, and Bill Pearl were noted for their massiveness in this area.

There is not a great deal you can do with the natural shape of the forearms. Some men like Casey Viator and Tim Belknap have lower arms that start almost at the base of the hand and immediately sweep into rotund elegance. Others have "long" wrists, almost entirely devoid of muscle until well along near the elbow. Al Beckles of London, England, is an example of this "Indian Club" phenomenon.

Because the forearms are in virtually constant use and have therefore developed a resistance to moderate exercise, they should be worked hard and with a system of high (10–20) repetitions. However, subjecting your forearms to progressive training is even more important than the repetition count. You will get nowhere by simply performing a few wrist or reverse curls at the end of your arm workout. You have to attack your forearms with a planned campaign of ever-increasing workloads. Then you will reap the rewards of your disciplined endeavor.

The incredible forearm of Tim Belknap.

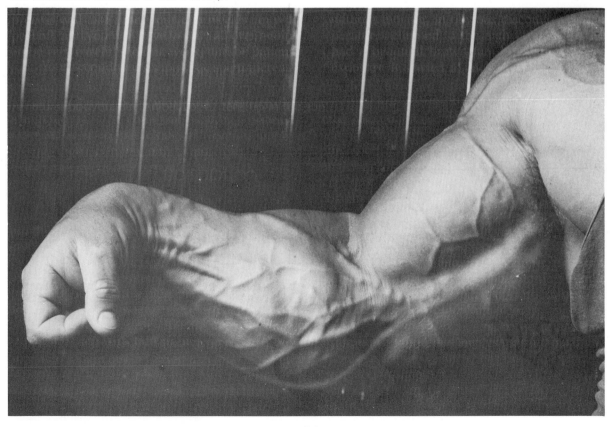

Wrist Curl

Wrist curls work the flexors (the belly) of the forearm. Perform them in a seated position, with your lower arms resting on your knees (palms up) or on the top of a bench. Your hands must be free. Arnold Schwarzenegger keeps his elbows close, while other stars allow their elbows to be comfortably apart—anything from 12–18 inches (30–45 cm).

Moving only your wrist, curl the weight upwards until your forearm is fully contracted. Allow the barbell to lower under control and you may (like Schwarzenegger and Draper) allow your fingers to "unroll" to some extent, but this is optional.

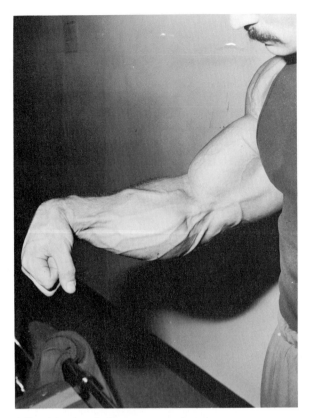

Mike Mentzer's forearm massiveness.

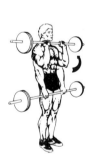

Reverse Curl

Stand erect, holding a barbell at slightly more than shoulder width. Allow the arms to hang down straight, elbows at your side, hands overgripped (knuckles up). As you curl the barbell, keep your wrists straight and level with your forearms and keep your elbows tucked in. Then lower, and repeat. You will feel this exercise in the upper forearm, near the elbow.

Reverse Wrist Curl

This exercise is performed in the same manner as the regular wrist curl, but your palms should face downwards instead of upwards. Also, you will be able to use less than half the weight in the reverse wrist curl. Most people find it more comfortable to keep the arms at least 12 inches (30 cm) apart in this variation.

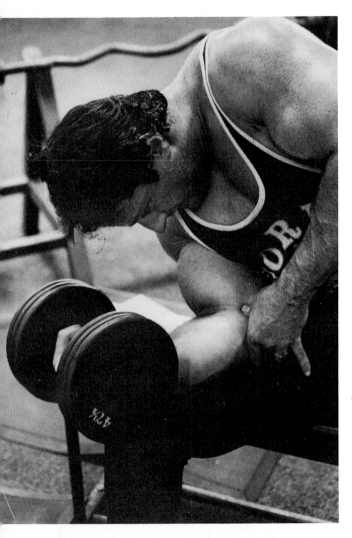

Rocky DeFerro does his wrist curls one arm at a time for ultra concentration.

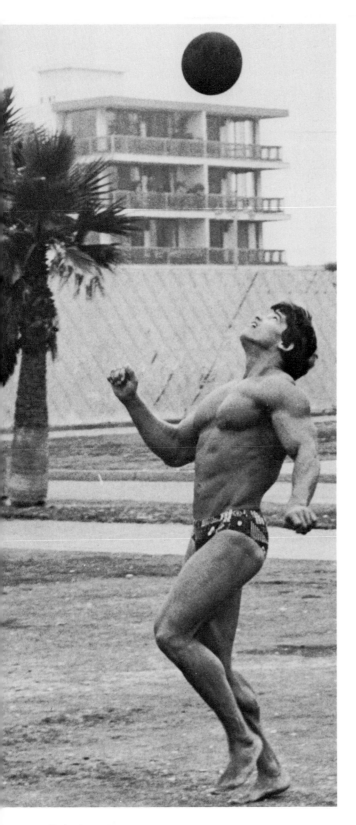

Enjoying himself in the sun—Arnold Schwarzenegger.

24

TANNING UP
Natural and Artificial Ways to Jack Up Your Tan

It is every bodybuilder's dream to someday stand on stage huge, ripped, and tanned. Yes, a glorious golden tan is as important as the development of a championship physique. Those two go hand in hand to achieve that look of super health and condition. How many times have you attended a physique competition where some fine physiques are completely unimpressive because they lack a tan? One almost turns his head in disgust as our would-be champion flexes and squeezes to show off his larva-white physique. Without a golden tan, our friend's chances of taking home a trophy are slim.

Many circumstances must be considered in our search for the ultimate tan. Sunlight could be considered the most important aspect of tanning, but it would be quite unfair to write a chapter on tanning without including the alternative sources of coloring. I will therefore discuss the natural as well as the artificial methods of acquiring a tan.

In dealing with natural sunlight one must be first warned that it can be very dangerous. The seriousness and pain of overexposure cannot be stressed enough. We have all gone through the ugly scene of waking up painfully burned after a few hours in the sun the day before. Some people are even foolish enough to go back into the sun in that condition. This is complete insanity. The additional exposure could land you in hospital.

There is absolutely no way that a tan can be rushed. The tan is Nature's way of protecting you from ultraviolet radiation, and it can't be obtained in a couple of lengthy exposures.

Your Skin

The skin consists of two layers which are separated by a thin membrane. The deeper layer, or *dermis*, is made up of blood and lymph vessels, fibrous tissue, sweat glands, hair follicles, and nerve endings. The outer layer, or *epidermis*, consists of a layer of basal cells that divide and form a top layering of squamous cells. In a continual process, squamous cells die and produce the *keratin layer*, the outermost protective coating which is ultimately sloughed off as a dandruff. The epidermis also contains *melanocytes*, cells that synthesize melanin pigment when exposed to ultraviolet radiation and produce the much sought-after tan.

Tanning is the skin's response to ultraviolet injury and its attempt to protect itself from further damage. It is like drawing the drapes in order to protect your system from too much light, but the body needs time to react efficiently. Each time you expose yourself to ultraviolet radiation, it has to synthesize the melanin pigment that produces the tan.

Sunburn is only the initial damage caused by ultraviolet radiation. Prolonged exposure to ultraviolet rays will also interfere with the production of collagen fibres in the dermis, causing the skin to lose elasticity and creating premature wrinkles. Further deterioration of the skin's outer layer deprives the epidermis of nutrition and leads to atrophy of the skin, which is another name for aging. Finally, with increased injury over a number of years of sunbathing, the ultimate price of your tan could be skin cancer.

It is not my intention to discourage any bodybuilder from sunbathing to acquire a tan, but I must warn you to use caution. It serves no purpose to sit in the sun all day in the hope of acquiring a darker tan. Skin cancer can be avoided with a dose of common sense. You must appraise your skin type and determine what sort of complexion you have. Not all people can handle a lot of sun; and yes, there are the unfortunate few who will never tan, no matter how long they expose themselves. As with everything else, genetics plays a big part. Fair people with blue eyes cannot hope to obtain as dark a tan as someone who has dark hair and eyes.

Remember that a sunburn can also throw you off schedule, since the skin must heal before it can be exposed again. After many years of burning and peeling, I finally realized that if you want a good tan, you must be patient and satisfied with what Nature has given you. Being fair-skinned, I can't hope to obtain a deep-brown tan. God knows, I suffered enough before realizing this fact. However, almost everyone can tan to some extent. Since I learned how to avoid sunburn, I have managed to get a reddish-brown tan.

Sensible Sunbathing

If you have a contest coming up, you should begin your exposure two or three weeks before the date of the contest. At the beginning, each exposure should be timed with care.

Before going into the sun, always apply a sunscreen to your lips and nose. I would also recommend that at this time you remove all body hair. This will give you an idea of how you are tanning. Certain areas can sometimes be very hard to judge if they are covered with lots of hair. Protect your eyesight by never looking directly into the sun. Ultraviolet radiation can severely injure the eyes.

Your first day of exposure should be no longer than 15–20 minutes front and back. I do not recommend any lotion which will allow you to stay in the sun any longer than the prescribed time. These lotions are advertised as containing sun-blocking agents which allow only the tanning rays to come through, but in my many years of tanning I have never found this to be true. I have never tanned any darker by using these special lotions. I don't believe that any kind of lotion can improve your skin color—unless it contains a dye. Use a sunscreen on your body if you wish to spend extra time swimming or playing in the sun without burning. However, this additional, screened exposure to the rays will not provide a deeper tan. Like everything else, your rate of tanning is dependent on genetics.

I might also mention that you can use a lotion or oil that has no sunscreen. This will provide a bit of welcome moisture for the skin, which can get very dry from the sun.

After the first day, study your body closely to see how your skin reacted to your first exposure. If you haven't burned, then increase your exposure to 30 minutes per side on the second day. You will probably find that 30 minutes will cause you to redden a bit. It will take about three or four days at 30 minutes before you can increase the exposure. After four days, your skin will probably start to turn reddish-brown. The body's defenses have been mobilized into producing melanin pigment as a reaction to the sun's rays.

The final days of your first week's sunbathing should be spent in caution. This is a crucial time when you can burn, which will set you back weeks. If you think 30 minutes is not enough and suddenly go for 45, the result could be painful in more ways than one. If you burn, you have severely injured your skin. The healing process will take time. Your first week's tan will peel off, and you will have to start all over again. So be very careful the first week, and be patient!

Your second week should be spent increasing your time by 5–10 minute doses, so by the end of two weeks, your exposure will be 60 minutes per side.

After two weeks, you should have a good base tan. The degree of your tan will depend on your complexion and genetics.

With two weeks of exposure under your belt, you can now decide where you want to go from here. I feel that it serves no purpose to spend hours in the sun. It has been my experience that regardless how long you now expose yourself, you will not improve on this tan. If a contest is near, then you might go for an hour and a half per side, but only for a week or so before the show. Once you have your tan, you can keep it golden by spending only one hour sunbathing two or three times a week. The dangers of hours upon hours of exposure have been spelled out earlier. I remember a rather attractive young woman I used to notice at the beach. I was on vacation, and she must have been off for the summer, because I saw her spread flat on a beach blanket every day. She would just lie there without moving, in obvious discomfort as temperatures climbed to the high 80's. At first she had a beautiful brown tan, but with increased exposure it started to look grey. Her exposure

A natural bodybuilder, Anibal Lopez tans up in the sun.

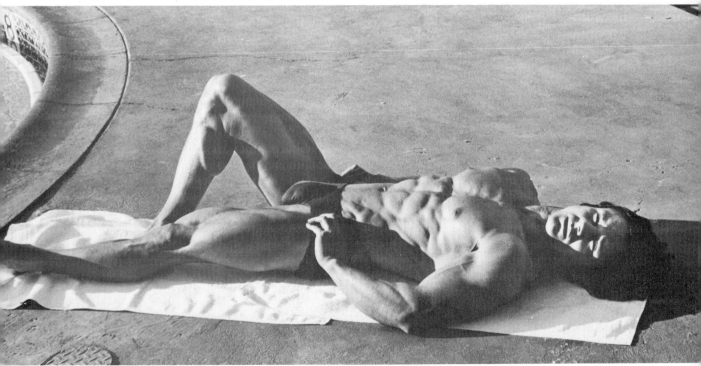

137

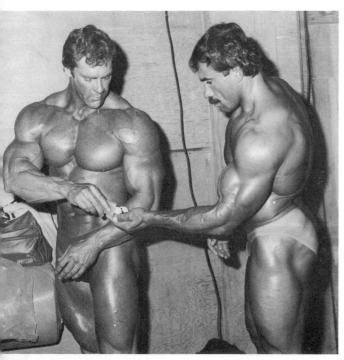
Pro champs Scott Wilson and Ali Mala believe in maximum sun-tanning.

each day was five and six hours, and this must have gone on all summer, because after I'd gone back to work, I still went to the beach on weekends, and sure enough, she was there. My final encounter with this poor soul came late that summer when I was shopping at a local mall. I walked into a clothing store, and there before my eyes was the sunworshipper I had watched all summer. She did not have a healthy glow. She looked much older, and her skin was dry, flaccid, and dark grey. That's what the excess exposure to ultraviolet rays had done to her.

In summary: the sun is a very dangerous friend. You will accomplish nothing by spending hour after hour broiling in its intense rays. Even moderate exposure will leave you weak and listless, making it hard to train with your usual intensity. Unfortunately, competing without a beautiful tan is like trying to run a mile with only one leg.

Who Needs More Than Sunshine?

It may come as a surprise to the natives of California and Florida, but 90 percent of the people in North America live in a climate where the sun is available to them only five to six months of the year. This leaves us northerners at an extreme disadvantage come contest time. In many cases a lot of our contests are in the spring, fall, or winter months. We are therefore left with the dilemma of finding a source of tanning other than a $2,000 trip to the south. Fortunately, there is a variety of artificial aids that allow the competing bodybuilder to obtain a less expensive tan.

Suntan Lamps

Suntan lamps fall into two categories: expensive and inexpensive. The inexpensive lamps can be purchased from almost any department store. The advertisements call them "the answer to that winter whiteness," and they go on to say that you can sport a glorious tan all winter if you purchase one. Sadly, I have never found this to be a fact. In my experience, they have been liberal on burning and conservative with tanning. Yes, you will obtain a little color from them, but it tends to go to the far side of red, rather than brown. People with darker complexions than mine may get better results from them.

If you do plan on using a sunlamp, then be extra careful regarding exposure. The rays from these lamps are very concentrated, and very few extra minutes of exposure can leave you severely burned. Read the instructions that come with the unit very carefully, and follow them to the letter. I have found suntan lamps useful for obtaining a little exposure before I go on a vacation and out into the sun. It allows the body to accustom itself to natural sunlight faster. So while these inexpensive lamps will not give you a glorious tan, they'll give you some color, and that is better than nothing.

The expensive lamps can be found in the now very popular tanning salons. It seems that a lot of research has been done for these artificial tanning booths. The first results were not that good, but recent advances in technique have produced lamps that really work. They are advertised as providing rays that tan without burning. However, if you burn easily in natural sunlight, then these lamps will burn you also. So the value of these expensive salons will depend on your complexion. Discussing their merits with some of our pro bodybuilders, I was told that they do work. The only drawback is that the tan they give you will fade much sooner than a natural tan. Still, they can be of great benefit to a competing bodybuilder.

For anyone using these salons for a number of visits, the system of tanning and the exposure time will be determined by the host of the salon, who starts people off with a brief exposure and then increases the exposures until a tan results. These visits may cover a period of months. The only complaint I have is that everyone is treated the same. In most cases, a person with a dark complexion can handle much more sun than someone with a fair complexion.

Tanning Pills

In theory, when you swallow these pills you tan from the inside out. They come under many brand names, one of the most popular being Orobronze. These pills contain a synthetic canthaxanthin, a coloring agent found naturally in certain crustaceans, fish, feathers, and vegetables. Through these pills, your skin will take on a shade of orange-brown that varies according to skin type. The pills are harmless and tend to work best in combination with natural sun.

The usual dose depends on the person's weight, surface area, and his ability to assimilate this substance. It usually takes fifteen days for an individual to show a color change, which peaks in twenty days. Don't expect too much. This sort of tan does not look natural, and it can leave you as orange as a carrot. Your color will not change drastically as a rule, just to a light orange, but in combination with natural sunlight, the pills can produce quite spectacular results.

One drawback of taking these tanning pills can be bright orange palms. For some reason the palms of your hands seem to pick up more color than the rest of your body, and that can look rather amusing.

Bronzing Lotions

The most popular means of obtaining an artificial tan is probably the use of tanning lotions. Many such products are on the market, and Sudden Tan™ by Coppertone™ is one of the most popular. The results of these lotions depend on brand, skin type, and how well they are applied. I have often seen pro bodybuilders who had the stuff smeared all over them unevenly; so they looked terrible and blotchy. Some had it mixed with oil, which made some areas run more than others, and that gave them a patchy appearance with certain parts of the body

To stand out on stage at a physique event, one must be really well tanned. (Left to right) Rory Leidelmeyer, Ray Boone, Tim Belknap, Bronston Austin, Jr.

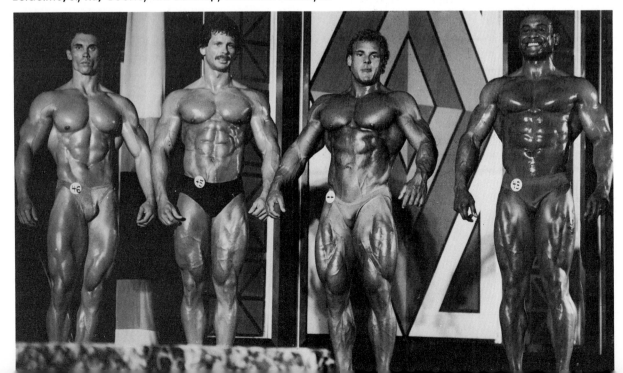

whiter than others. This sort of thing should be avoided at all costs.

The secret of applying a good coating of suntan lotion is patience. If you have a contest coming up on Saturday, apply your first coating early Friday morning. Your first coat should be light, and I do not believe in rubber gloves or a sponge. There is nothing like the sensitive palms of your hands for applying a good even coating of Sudden Tan. Don't use a lot. Just rub a little on each body part and rub it in evenly. Rub very little on your knees or elbow joints, for they tend to absorb more than the rest of the body, and don't apply any to the face this first time. As soon as you have rubbed a light coating all over your body, including the back, just rest and let it dry. Do nothing that might cause you to sweat, or else the tanning lotion might run.

One point to remember is that your color will be much better if you can get some natural sun in addition. But even a lamp or a salon will improve the result.

With the first coat applied early in the morning, apply the second coating about mid-afternoon. Include the face, but otherwise follow the same procedure: very light, even applications to each body part. Under no circumstances try to apply a lot of lotion in an effort to obtain an immediate tan. It may take several light applications before you finally notice your skin taking on any color. The final coat on Friday should be applied just before going to bed. Use the same methodical procedure. A little on the arms, rub it in, then on the chest and stomach. Each area must be completely rubbed in before you go on to another.

The morning of the contest, you will find that your skin has taken on a fairly good color. The degree of the browning effect will vary from individual to individual, depending on the skin type. Some people will get quite brown, while others tend to go orange. The day of the contest you should try to apply two more coats. One early in the morning, and the second just before contest time. Any further coats of this Sudden Tan lotion will not give you a better tan. They would just give you a fake look and tend to shade your cuts.

One of the most worst mistakes that many bodybuilders have made before a contest is to rub oil over the tanning lotion on their body before going on stage. Often the artificial tan will run with the oil and give the contestant a most unflattering appearance. Even some of our top pros fall prey to this situation, so be very careful about selecting a gloss you rub on in conjunction with a fake tan. Arnold was known to apply a light coat of Nivea cream before going on stage. Oil does give you better highlights, however. If you use it, make sure it is compatible with your artificial tanning lotion.

Conclusion

I have found that nothing can replace a good natural tan obtained over a period of weeks. The next best thing is a combination of Orobronze, sunlamp, and Sudden Tan. In achieving a good color for a competition, the most important factors are patience and moderation.

By following the advice I have given you in this chapter, you can get yourself the best tan of your life, and that will certainly give you an edge in the competition. If you are not competing, your golden, even tan will make you look fantastic just the same. But remember, *patience*!

Points to Remember

• After sunbathing, always apply a good coating of skin moisturizing cream to replace the natural oils lost during exposure.
• Your face may not be able to stand as much exposure as your body, so limit the direct exposure of your face.
• Always apply a screening agent to the extra sensitive areas such as the lips, nose, and all around the edges of your swimming trunks.
• To obtain an even tan, remember to expose the under-arm areas as well as the rest of the body.
• Turn your blanket or chair in the direction of the sun so that the direct rays will fall on you evenly.
• Be aware that sand and water reflect ultraviolet light and thus increase its intensity.
• A hazy or cloudy day does not necessarily allow you a longer exposure time. The ultraviolet rays may filter through and burn you all the same.
• Be careful of sunstroke. Burning is not the only danger of spending too much time in the sun.
• You will become dehydrated from perspiration, so drink plenty of fluids (low in sugar).

25 ROUTINES FOR ADDING SIZE
Maxing Out the Muscle

Lee Haney, a Mr. America with everything.

I have written several bodybuilding books to date, scores of courses and manuals, and literally hundreds of articles. Many of them did not exactly set the bodybuilding world on fire. The first indication that somebody was reading even one word of my writings came after I'd written an article for Bob Hoffman's *Muscular Development* magazine. The title of the piece was *Where Are We Heading?* and it dealt with the oncoming mania of drug-taking in the sport. That was way back in the 60's, and *Muscular Development's* editor John Grimek told me that it brought more response from readers than any other article he could remember. Every few days I would get bundles of letters sent on to me. Most were in agreement with my views. A few disagreed.

A couple of years later I conceived the idea of *pre-exhaust*. I tried it out on myself and a few members of the gym I was training at, and found that I really seemed to have hit on to something. I wrote up the principle for *Iron Man Magazine* in 1968, but didn't realize the huge impact the system carried until Nautilus inventor Arthur

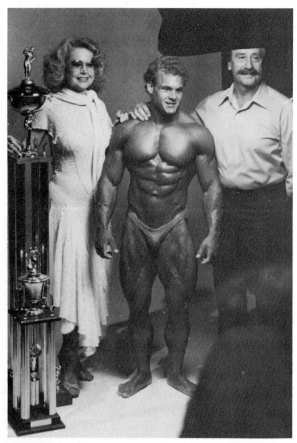

Betty and Joe Weider pose for the *Muscle and Fitness* cameras with Mr. America Tim Belknap.

I resisted the advice of my accountant to bankrupt the magazine, and am very glad I did. While we were sinking because of cash-flow problems, Joe Weider, whom I regard as nothing less than a publishing genius, drew on his access to huge financial resources, doubled the page size in his own magazine (known as *Musclebuilder* in those days), went "all color," and consequently took back his place at the top of the muscle publishing industry. His magazine, now known as *Muscle and Fitness*, leads the world in quality and sales. But little old *MuscleMag International* is in there, a satisfying and solid second, as an all-training magazine.

Then came *Hardcore Bodybuilding*. The initial sales were tremendous, and it is still being bought in book stores the world over. With the advent of *Hardcore*, I was asked to appear on numerous radio and TV talk shows, and my mail, already heavy from response to my writing in *MuscleMag*, has doubled.

Perhaps this background sketch of my life in the world of bodybuilding is boring. I am *sure* it is boring. But I bring it to your attention in the faint hope that you will consider the possibility that when it comes to bodybuilding, I may, at least to a small degree, know what I am talking about.

No, I am *not* the world's top expert in bodybuilding. I can think of many more knowledgeable than myself. But I *am* involved with the sport on a daily basis, and I *do* continue to train. So why am I a bodybuilding failure? Why does Bob Kennedy, author and publisher of so much bodybuilding information, not have 22-inch arms and a 55-inch chest? The answer is simple. No matter what I do, did, or will do, it just won't happen. Maybe if I had resorted to steroids (which I never did because of outright fear) I would have taken my arms from 18 inches to 19. So what! The truth is, with the skinniest father imaginable, I just wasn't handed down the genes for greatness. I mention all this because, hell of all hells, *you* may be in the same boat!

Training at Home

The overriding question I get asked both by beginners and advanced bodybuilders involves the training routine. Everybody, it seems, wants to train with a routine that offers the maximum amount of return for time and energy spent.

Jones incorporated the pre-exhaust ideas into many of his machines. This was a brilliant move on his part because, even today, it sets his machines apart from all the others, most of them little more than crude imitations. To his credit, Jones didn't claim to have invented the pre-exhaust system but openly acknowledged my article. Of course he, and he alone, ultimately developed this concept into his excellent line of Nautilus equipment.

The next step up in my life came when I introduced my own bodybuilding publication, *MuscleMag International*, to the world. It quickly became the best selling bodybuilding publication of all. We introduced color pictures inside the mag at a time when everyone else was running black-and-white only. Unfortunately, even though our sales were good, I found myself floundering in a sea of problems. *MuscleMag* was costing more to produce than we were getting back in sales.

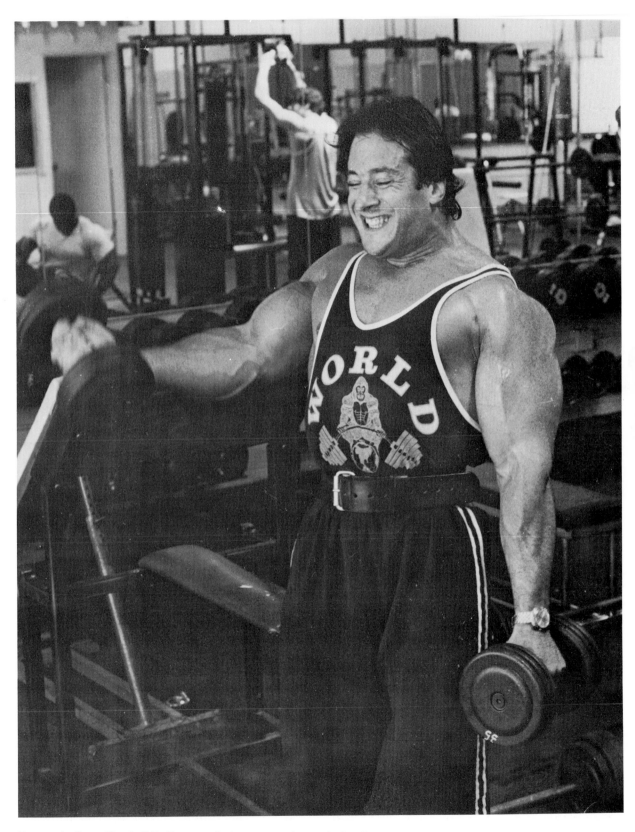

To watch Greg "Rocky" DeFerro train is an experience in itself.

Let me deal first with the home trainer who has limited facilities to train with. He probably has no lat machine, leg press, or leg extension apparatus. Pek-Deks and scott curl bench are beyond his financial reach. But here are some things you simply *must* acquire, even if you have to make them yourself!

First, you should have a flat bench with weight support stands. All the better if it is an adjustable flat/incline bench, but certainly a basic flat bench is *essential*. The only other absolute *must* is a pair of squat stands. These can be bought for under $100, but many youngsters have been able to make their own squat stands out of wood, or got a friend or relation to make a set for them. The point to bear in mind is that without these important training aids you can't really progress in either the squat or the bench press, both of them standard basic exercises. Needless to say, you will also need a 6-foot (110 cm) bar and a pair of 16-inch (40 cm) dumbbell rods, and enough weight discs to challenge you in the heaviest exercises.

Here is a very good, proven beginner's routine that will get you growing and keep you growing for some time. Do not make the mistake of thinking that more is necessarily better. More people have gained more muscle on *abbreviated* weight programs than on any other system. This last sentence is so important, I want you to read it again. *More people have gained more muscle on abbreviated weight programs than on any other system.*

Basic Routine

Warm-Up	1 minute rope jumping
Press Behind Neck	3 × 8
Squat	3 × 10
Bench Press	3 × 8
Bent-Over Rowing	3 × 10
Calf Raise	3 × 25
Barbell Curl	3 × 10
Triceps Stretch	3 × 12
Sit-ups	3 × 20

Incredibly, the above schedule can prove super effective for even the intermediate or advanced bodybuilder, at least for a 3–6 month period. You will, of course, make better progress if you have a calf raise machine for calf work in the above schedule. If you do not have access to one, then do the next best thing: hold a loaded barbell across the back of your shoulders for added resistance.

The next routine I'm going to give you is a special schedule, called the super routine, for the more advanced trainer. This routine has been around for some time and is extremely popular.

The Super Routine

Warm-up	Rope Skipping, 200–300 jumps
Shoulders	
Seated Press Behind Neck	4 × 8–10
NonStop Dumbbell Raises:	
forward, side, and bent over	3 × 10 each
Upright rowing	4 × 8–12
Thighs	
Front Squat	
(heels on 3-inch wood block)	5 × 8–12
Hack Lift	3 × 10–12
Thigh Curls	3 × 10–15
Chest	
Wide-Grip Bench Press to upper	
sternum	6 × 6–12
Incline Dumbbell Bench Press	
(45-degree angle)	4 × 10–12
Back	
Prone Hyperextensions	3 × 10–20
Wide-Grip Chin Behind Neck	4 × 10–15
Single Dumbbell Rowing	4 × 8–12
Calves	
Heel Raise	
(block, but no weight)	4 × 15–25
Donkey Calf Raise	4 × 15–30

For those who wish to split this routine, it is advocated that you split it so as to train six days a week and rest one. You could, for example, divide as follows:

Monday, Wednesday, Friday
Shoulders
Chest
Neck and Traps
Triceps
Tuesday, Thursday, Saturday
Thighs
Back
Calves
Forearms
Abs
Biceps

Magic Schedules

It would be quite wrong for any physical training instructor to infer that there is only one way to acquire a good physique. There are many different methods, and not all of them involve the use of barbell and dumbbells. Wrestling, hand balancing, weight lifting, and gymnastics all add greatly to the musculature. It is undisputed, however, that the best methods involve the use of progressive resistance, but within this category, no single routine can truthfully be called "the best." There is *no* magic schedule by which rapid gains can be secured or guaranteed with certainty.

Too many bodybuilders are waiting for this *one* schedule to be divulged. However, it just does not exist.

By and large, bodybuilders are willing to do almost anything to accelerate their muscle growth. Thus I would not hesitate to recommend any type of training madness if I thought it would help you get where you want to go. (Note, I said training madness, not steroid madness.)

I myself have done a heavy set of curls, 10 repetitions every half hour from 9 AM until 9 PM, making a total of 24 all-out sets, in order to "shock" my biceps into growing. The result was a tumultuous headache the next day and very sore swollen biceps that appeared at first to have grown, but eventually diminished to their original 15¼ inches.

I have trained the entire body every day for a month with little change. On another occasion I did 50 sets of calf raises in three hours and spent a week in bed!

I tell you all this in an effort to convince you that my thoughts are in no way conservative where bodybuilding is concerned. Because I know that you are looking for the best musclebuilding techniques, I would not hestitate to recommend *any* exercise procedure to you if I thought it would work, even if the results were disproportionately small to the effort involved. But the truth is they don't work.

The Tough Old Days

Few people realize that on the whole the old-time bodybuilders trained far harder than the musclemen of today. Talking with Armand Tanny, a former Mr. USA and a very knowledge-able man on matters of muscle, he related how, in the golden days of Muscle Beach, it was quite common for him and his training partners to train *all day long* and think nothing of it.

He and his training buddies would do sets of repetition bench presses or curls that went on for hour after hour, from morning till dusk. One man, Zabo Koszewski, wouldn't even start his workout until he had done 1,000 sit-ups plus 1,000 leg raises! The 1951 Mr. America, Roy Hilligen, would do four hours of squats, plus another four hours of presses, and then he'd go on to finish his workout.

John Grimek, never a man to take the easy path, would do anything to get bigger. He has been observed performing scores of sets of just

Tom Platz.

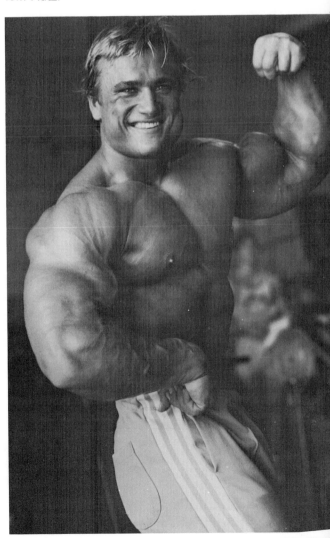

one exercise, and at one time he was doing repetition free squats every workout. He performed thousands of nonstop repetitions!!

The Deep-Knee-Bend System and Beyond

A more moderate routine that received a great deal of publicity in the magazines of the day and was rightly considered to be the superior system of the day was the Deep-Knee-Bend System for gaining muscular bodyweight. An examination of its development is worthwhile.

The value of this routine consisted of a few exercises for the large muscle groups. It was first mentioned nearly sixty years ago in George F. Jowett's book, *Key to Might and Muscle*. At that time, the average program consisted of at least 12 exercises, and sometimes 20 or more. It was not until 1930 or thereabouts that Mark H. Berry, editor of *Strength* magazine, began to appreciate the possibilities of a shorter type of routine with an enormous emphasis upon heavy leg work. Berry was greatly impressed by Henry Steinborn, the top class pro wrestler and weight lifter of the era. Steinborn had accomplished an "impossible" 370 clean and jerk and had performed an incredible number of heavy squats in

Lou Ferrigno at World's Gym—a photo session for the Weider publications before he leaves for Italy to film "Hercules."

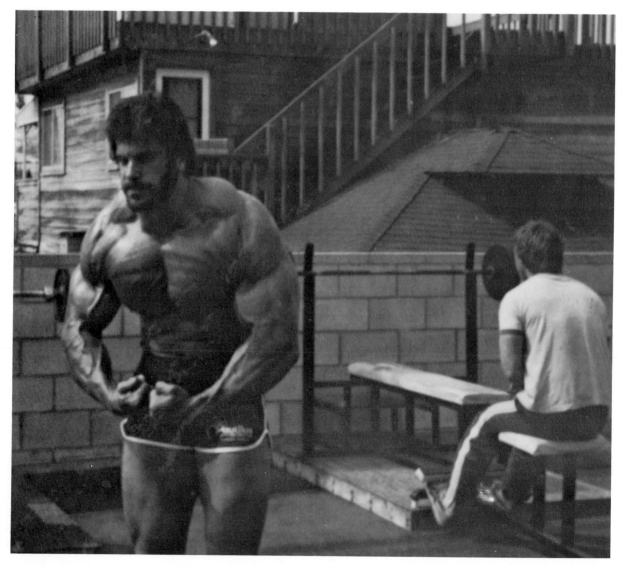

146

the course of his training at Sig Klein's barbell studio in New York.

When Mark Berry found out about Steinborn's training, he recommended similar training to other weightlifters for improving their leg strength and lifting ability. Rather to Berry's surprise, many students who took his advice began to report gains in bodyweight. This encouraged Berry to make further experiments.

Strength magazine had a wide distribution, so the deep-knee-bend method of increasing weight very soon became a standard method. Pupils all over the world tried it and made excellent gains. This led Mark Berry to conclude that the deep knee bend (squat) and other heavy exercises were stimulating to the system. Then a method was devised which used no isolation exercises (minor movements). The basic routine that proved helpful to many barbell men of the day was:

> Press Behind Neck
> Squat (Deep Knee Bend)
> Two-Hands Standing Press
> Stiff-Legged Dead Lift
> Bench Press (Press on Back)

The three upper-body exercises were performed with one set each, 10–12 repetitions, and the deep knee bend and stiff-legged dead lift with 20 repetitions. The routine was to be performed three times a week, and no other exercise (such as abdominal work) was to be performed. Emphasis was placed on the importance of adequate food and rest.

John Grimek, *the* physique of the 40's, reportedly used Berry's routine with great success. Ultimately, *Strength* magazine went out of business, but a young and vigorous publisher named Peary Rader was ready to promote the Berry System through his writings. Rader had started a typewritten, multigraphed, bodybuilding bulletin and had managed to gain a core of enthusiastic subscribers. The name of his bulletin, soon to become a respected, fully fledged magazine was *Iron Man*.

With constant feedback from his readers, and in consultation with deep-knee-bend exponents Roger Eells and Jose Hise (who gained 29 pounds in one month with the Deep-Knee-Bend System), Rader came up with a revised routine, which omitted the stiff-legged dead lift but included the rowing motion, the straight-arm pullover, and the two-hand curl.

Peary Rader's Routine

Press Behind Neck	3 sets of 8 reps
Squat	
(*alternating with*)	3 sets of 20 reps
Straight Arm Pullover	
Bench Press	3 sets of 8 reps
Barbell Curl	3 sets of 8 reps

Multi-Poundage

Following on from the Rader System, the British magazine *Vigor* came out with a useful program promoted under the name of *The Atkin Multi-Poundage System*. Like all other systems, it aimed to maximize gains in the shortest possible time, and it was widely practiced throughout the world.

Here is how it was set up:

The basic idea behind this multi-poundage system was to keep a muscle group working against maximum poundage throughout any number of repetitions. In a normal system (as opposed to a multi-poundage system) a bodybuilder does not feel the weight until the last few repetitions. Atkin felt this to be a waste. Accordingly, his system (sometimes called *triple-dropping*) let a trainer start his set with a heavy weight. After a few repetitions, two discs would be removed. After another few repetitions, a further weight reduction was made.

When you first use this technique it is a good idea to reduce the weight when you feel you could perform a couple more reps. Later, as proficiency becomes evident, you can push until you cannot perform another rep. Incidentally, this method is definitely *not* for beginners.

When you apply this principle to dumbbell training, have one or two pairs of lighter dumbbells ready to use as you train. Then, when you can't go on pressing a pair of fifty-pounders, lower them to the ground, and quickly pick up a pair of forty-pounders. For the last few repetitions, you can replace them with a pair of thirty-pounders and train with those until you cannot do another rep.

It doesn't matter how you break up a set. Some people use a system of $3 \times 3 \times 3$ to make a set of 9 reps. Others work with $5 \times 5 \times 5$ to make a set of 15 reps. Needless to say, this method, especially when using barbells, is not suited to the lone home trainer. You need assistance from two workout partners, one on either side of your exercise bar, to slip off a disc every few reps as you progress through your set.

Training in the 1950's

In the 1950's Reg Park came to the fore in the world of physiques. Reg, at 6 feet 1.5 inches, was 240 pounds of bone and muscle and made *every* other bodybuilder in the world look small beside him, clothed or unclothed.

His training routine, too, was influenced by the deep-knee-bend phenomenon. Many thousands of weight men were influenced by Reg's training system, which was highly publicized in the *Reg Park Journal* he published as a monthly in Britain. The program below, which the many-time Mr. Universe winner used when going for maximum size, is a limited program. Park, who trained with hundreds of different exercise variations in his career, is now in his mid-fifties and still considers it one of the best systems. Reg often split this routine in two and trained five or six days a week.

Reg Park's Routine

Prone Hyper Extensions	5 × 10
Press Behind Neck	5 × 8
Seated Dumbbell Press	5 × 8
Squat	5 × 8
Hack Squats	5 × 10
Bench Press	5 × 6
Flying Exercise	5 × 10
Rowing	5 × 8
Chin Behind Neck	5 × 12
Barbell Curl	5 × 8
Incline Dumbbell Curl	5 × 8
Lying Triceps Curl	5 × 10
Dumbbell Triceps Extensions	5 × 12

At around the same time Park was training, Steve Reeves, whose good looks and super proportions appealed to not only bodybuilders but to the general public, was working out in a slightly different way. He trained the whole body three days a week, with a day's rest between each workout.

Actually, Steve trained very hard, with a Mentzer-like intensity, often performing negatives. For example, if while performing the incline dumbbell curls he could not get the weight up, he would assist with his leg by kicking the weight up, and would then concentrate on

lowering the dumbbell slowly. Because Reeves used such high intensity he seldom found it necessary to perform more than 3 sets of any exercise. Steve liked variety in his training, so he would frequently change his routine around.

Steve Reeves' Routine

Upright Rowing	3 × 9
Press Behind Neck	3 × 9
Lateral Raise	3 × 10
Wide-Grip Bench Press	3 × 9
Incline Dumbbell Press	3 × 9
Flying	3 × 12
Chins Behind Neck	3 × 11
Seated Pulley Rowing	3 × 11
Decline Pullovers	3 × 11
Strict Incline Dumbbell Curls	8 × 5
Triceps Pressdowns	5 × 8
Single-Arm Lying Dumbbell Extensions	5 × 12
Barbell Squats	3 × 6
Front Squats	4 × 12
Leg Curls	3 × 12
Calf Raise	3 × 20

Longer Routines and Split Routines

Gradually, as bodybuilding contests became more popular throughout the 60's and 70's, people's routines became longer. It became common for serious bodybuilders to split their routines into two parts in order to shorten their training time.

Years ago virtually no one performed exercises for the small areas of the body. Thigh biceps, serratus, posterior delts, brachialis, rhomboids, erectors, teres, and tibialis were largely overlooked. Today we pay attention to developing the smaller muscles of the body, so the schedules of the champs tend to be longer. You as an aspiring bodybuilder should not try to emulate a champion bodybuilder's routine. Instead of gaining from it, you could easily tire yourself out completely.

Here, for example, is a typical Arnold Schwarzenegger routine. Bear in mind that Arnold frequently chopped and changed his exercises around "to keep my muscles guessing." Today, because Arnold does not compete anymore, he does much less. He is no longer motivated to build the huge 58-inch chest and

23-inch arms that brought him seven Mr. Olympia crowns and the title of World's Greatest Bodybuilder.

Arnold Schwarzenegger's Mr. Olympia Routine

Monday, Wednesday, Friday
Mornings
Chest

Bench press	5 × 8 to 10 reps
Flat Bench Flyes	5 × 8 reps
Incline Press	6 × 8–10 reps
Parallel Bar Dips (body weight)	5 sets
Cable Crossovers	6 sets × 12 reps
Dumbbell Pullover across Bench	5 × 10 reps

Back

Wide-Grip Chins to Front (body weight)	6 sets
T-Bar Rows	5 × 8 reps
Long Cable Pull	6 × 8 reps
Barbell Rows	6 × 12 reps
Hi-Rep Deadlifts on Box	6 × 15 reps
Single-Arm Dumbbell Row	5 × 8 reps

Upper Legs

Back Squats	6 × 10–12 reps
Leg Extensions	6 × 15 reps
Leg Press	6 × 8–10 reps
Leg Curls	6 × 12 reps
Barbell Lunges	5 × 15 reps

Afternoons
Calves

Heel Raise on Calf Machine	10 × 10 reps
Seated Heel Raise	8 × 15 reps
Single-Leg Heel Raise	6 × 12 reps

Forearms

Wrist Roller Curls	4 sets
Reverse Barbell Curl	4 × 8 reps
Wrist Curls	4 × 10 reps

Tuesday, Thursday, and Saturday
Arms

Cheat Barbell Curl	6 sets 8 reps
Seated Dumbbell Curl	6 sets 6 reps
Concentration Curl	6 sets 10 reps
Close-Grip Press	6 sets 8 reps
Triceps Pressdowns	6 sets 10 reps
Barbell French Presses	6 sets 8 reps
Single-Arm Triceps Stretch	6 sets 10 reps

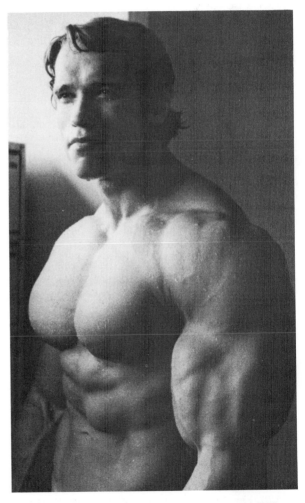

Arnold Schwarzenegger, who has won the IFBB Mr. Olympia a monumental 7 times, believes in shocking the muscles with constantly changing routines.

Shoulders

Seated Front Press	6 sets 8 to 10 reps
Standing Lateral Raise	6 sets 10 reps
Dumbbell Press	6 sets 8 reps
Seated Bent-Over Laterals	5 sets 10 reps
Cable Laterals	5 sets 12 reps

Calves

Heel Raise on Calf Machine	10×10 reps
Seated Heel Raise	8×15 reps
Single-Leg Calf Raise	6×12 reps

Forearms

Wrist Roller Curls	4 sets
Reverse Barbell Curl	4×8 reps
Wrist Curl	4×10 reps

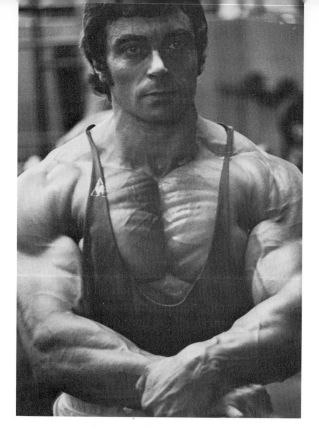

Frenchman Gerard Buinoud experiments for super size.

After examining Schwarzenegger's schedule, one could rightfully conclude that he does just about *everything*. Each muscle area is worked, and worked hard. Unlike Mike Mentzer, Arnold attributes his success to the concept of practicing "plenty of sets and reps."

Your Own Routine

Unless you are a very advanced bodybuilder, you won't be able to gain by using that schedule of Arnold Schwarzenegger's. You will have to tailor his ideas and exercises to your own physical condition. Instead of five or six exercises per bodypart, do two or three. You can add exercises as your body gains in strength and condition. The important thing to remember about a routine is that it must be *balanced*. You just cannot grow if you are not working *all* the muscles.

Many beginners avoid heavy leg work like the plague. Even if your legs are naturally well developed, you should still work them regularly. The same holds true for all basic body parts. They should be worked on a regular basis. Of course, your weakest areas should be worked the hardest.

Another thing to keep in mind is that a schedule is not some magic collection of secret movements. It is simply a collection of *workable exercises for increasing the size of your muscles*. You have to schedule exercises for each area and perform enough sets and reps to stimulate growth without inducing an overtrained condition. Far better to adopt a short routine and add to it as you progress in fitness and strength than to tackle an overlong routine, which will serve to dig you into a sticking point you'll never forget. Start with a limited program, and add, add, add as you grow, grow, grow.

It wouldn't be right to have a discourse on routines without mentioning the views of veteran bodybuilder Vince Gironda. (Vince will be working on a book with this author shortly.)

It almost seems that Vince, the Iron Guru, was the originator of the modern routine as we know it today. His ideas were always revolutionary, and even forty years ago he was ahead of his time.

Gironda cautions that beginners should start off with only 3 sets of 8 reps (most authorities feel that one or two sets is enough for beginners). "After the first month," says

Gironda, "I recommend that the beginner use 5 sets of 5 reps, the third month 6 sets of 6 reps and, ultimately, after the sixth month, the trainer should be trying the advanced '8 sets of 8 reps' routine."

Gironda, of course, has experimented with numerous, possibly thousands, of routines and their myriad variations. He has concluded that the seasoned bodybuilder can always get an *honest* workout by performing a routine (every other day) consisting of working one exercise per body part for 8 sets of 8 reps (except calves which Vince says are, "a *high rep* muscle, and 20 reps minimum should be employed.")

A typical Gironda workout schedule, which has proved itself successful time and time again at his North Hollywood gym, is as follows:

Dumbbell Lateral Raises	8×8
(Lateral Deltoid Head)	
Wide Grip Parallel Bar Dips	8×8
(Upper and Outer Pectoral Area)	
Seated Lat Pulley Machine Rowing	8×8
(Mid and Lower Lat Area)	
Kneeling Face Down Cradle Bench	
Triceps Pulley Extension	8×8
(Low, Middle and Outside Heads)	
Body Drag Barbell Curls	8×8
(Upper, Mid and Lower Biceps)	
Front heels on Block Squat	8×8
(Mid and Lower Thigh)	
Calf Raise	8×20
(Gastrocnemius)	
Crunches with Weight	8×8
(Upper and Lower Abdominals)	

Lance Dreher—his future is destined for greatness.

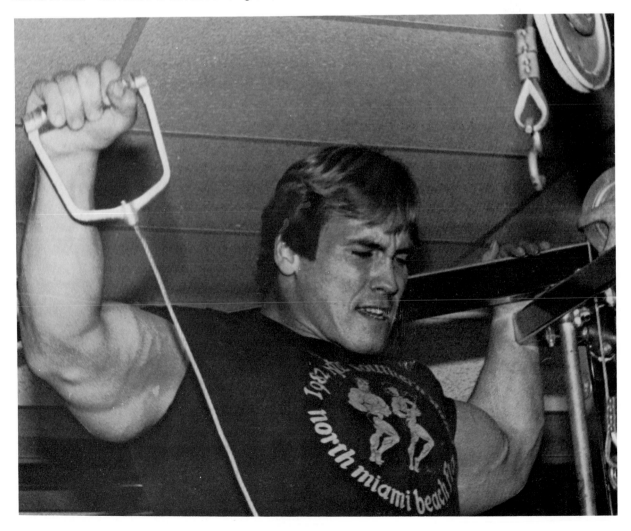

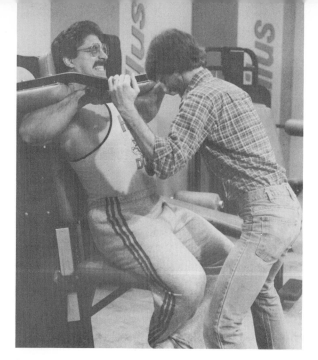

Roy Mentzer gets a little extra resistance for his Nautilus shoulder raises.

The question of tailoring your routine for your physical type has been mentioned earlier. Genetics determine whether you are a hard gainer or not. Bodybuilding champions like Larry Scott, Tony Pearson, and Frank Zane are considered hard gainers, while men like Tim Belknap, Lance Dreher, Scott Wilson, Casey Viator, and Mike Mentzer could be perceived as real "naturals" in the bodybuilding game. As author Bill Reynolds says: "It doesn't take a bodybuilder long to discover that some men make exceptionally fast gains while others make only mediocre or even slow progress."

Actually, being a slow gainer can be discouraging but quite often there is some compensation in the form of "natural" shape and contour. Joints, for example, are often smaller (neater) in the hard-gaining enthusiast and accordingly the muscles built around the wrists, elbows, ankles, knees look more impressive when contrasted with these more aesthetic bony areas.

The hard gainer's approach to bodybuilding has to be better planned, more scientific and orderly. He cannot get away with partying, smoking or boozing. His diet must be constantly at an optimum level, eating at times up to six to eight times a day (smaller quantities) to ensure that there is an ever-ready supply of nutrients for the body's needs.

If you are a hard gainer, then it will behoove you to limit the amount of exercises you do: never more than two for any single body part. Repetitions, too, should be curtailed, averaging around six and eight.

Here is a recommended hard gainers' off-season training routine.

Mondays and Thursdays
Shoulders

Press Behind Neck	4 × 6
Upright Rowing	4 × 8

Chest

Bench Press	6 × 6
Incline Flyes	4 × 8

Trapezius

Barbell Shrugs	4 × 5

Triceps

Parallel Bar Dips	5 × 6
Lying Triceps Stretch	5 × 8

Abdominals

Hanging Leg Raise	3 × 15

Tuesdays and Fridays
Upper Legs

Squat	5 × 6
Thigh Curls	3 × 10

Upper Back

Barbell Rows	4 × 6
Chin Behind Neck	4 × 8

Forearms

Reverse Curl	4 × 8

Lower Legs

Standing Calf Raise	4 × 20

Biceps

Barbell Curl	5 × 6
Inclining Dumbbell Curl	5 × 6

If you are ever fortunate enough to visit Gold's or World's gyms in Santa Monica, watch the top bodybuilders train. You'll be surprised—not by the unusual exercises they perform, but by the fact that they use all the usual movements. Virtually every bodybuilder of note uses: bench presses, flyes, squats, thigh extensions, thigh curls, presses behind neck, lateral raises, curls, triceps pressdowns, parallel bar dips, calf raises, chins, T-Bar rows, Roman chair sit-ups.

As a hopeful champion you can use these same basic exercises, tailor them to your own stage of development, and one day you'll get there!

26
TIPS TO BEAT OUT THE COMPETITION
The Winning Edge

Everybody knows the names of the top bodybuilders, men like Arnold Schwarzenegger, Franco Columbu, Sergio Oliva, Samir Bannout, Mohamed Makkawy, Boyer Coe. In fact, we know them so well, we don't even have to know their last names. All we need to hear is Arnold, Franco, Boyer, and we know exactly who's who.

But if you ever go to an amateur contest, especially at a national level, you will be awed by the number of really topflight physiques there are around. Thirty years ago, there were no more than a handful of men with 19-inch arms. Today, there are thousands upon thousands.

Yes, there is an abundance of really well-built guys around, yet there are not that many new faces breaking into the professional ranks. Of those who do, very few seem to be able to get their act together sufficiently to walk away with the top trophies.

It's a funny thing about bodybuilders—even the big-name professionals for the most part—when they fail to win a contest, they blame everyone else but themselves. If you've been to any seminars, you will know what I'm talking about. If that particular bodybuilder didn't win, he'll tell you that the decision was

Good sportsmanship. Fellow Brits Bertil Fox and Al Beckles shake hands before a posedown.

political. If he placed way down the list, he will claim the judges overlooked him and didn't compare him with the top men. I have heard many different bodybuilders claim this one, yet in reality they were not compared because they were totally out of it. They did not *merit* being compared. It would have been a waste of time.

What bodybuilders don't realize is that when they come out on stage and go through the relaxed and mandatory poses and what have you, they are being judged, scrutinized, and *compared* right there. Lack of size, proportion, muscularity is quickly noticed by an observant judge. A guy may look phenomenal in his bathroom mirror, but in the company of other top bodybuilders, his great physique may pale beside a super-great one.

I remember when Arnold Schwarzenegger first came to the States and entered the IFBB Pro Mr. Universe against Frank Zane. Frank beat him, and I wrote in *Iron Man* magazine that Arnold was undertanned and relatively smooth

when compared to Zane. This was way back in the late 60's.

A year after this contest, Chet Yorton held a party at his Malibu Beach home, and since I was in California at the time, he asked me along. Almost as soon as the beer was flowing, Arnold started to belabor me for writing that he was smooth and pale at this show. Nothing I could say would calm him down. He insisted that he was in fact better than Zane, and that Joe Weider had arranged things so that he, Arnold, would have to pay his dues before winning in the USA. He would not concede that Zane was better developed or better prepared.

Another year went by and I was again out with Arnold, this time at the Los Angeles sporting club, for dinner with Joe Weider. Had Arnold's ego relaxed sufficiently for him to concede defeat by Zane? No way! He even told Joe to his face that he had arranged the result because Joe "stood to make more money out of Zane winning." Joe just laughed at all this and told Arnold

The man has charisma. Bronston Austin, Jr., acknowledges the judge's score cards.

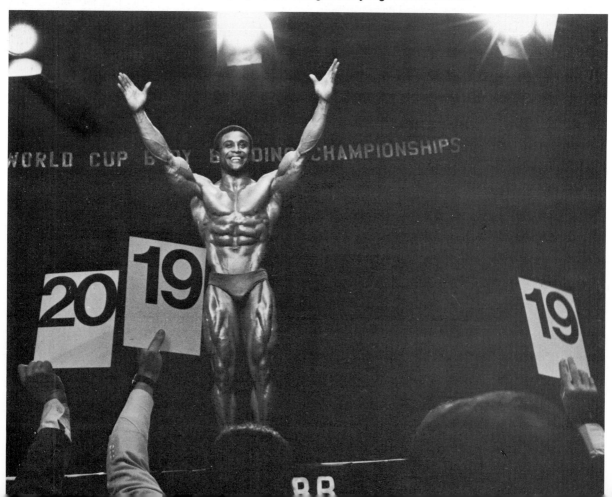

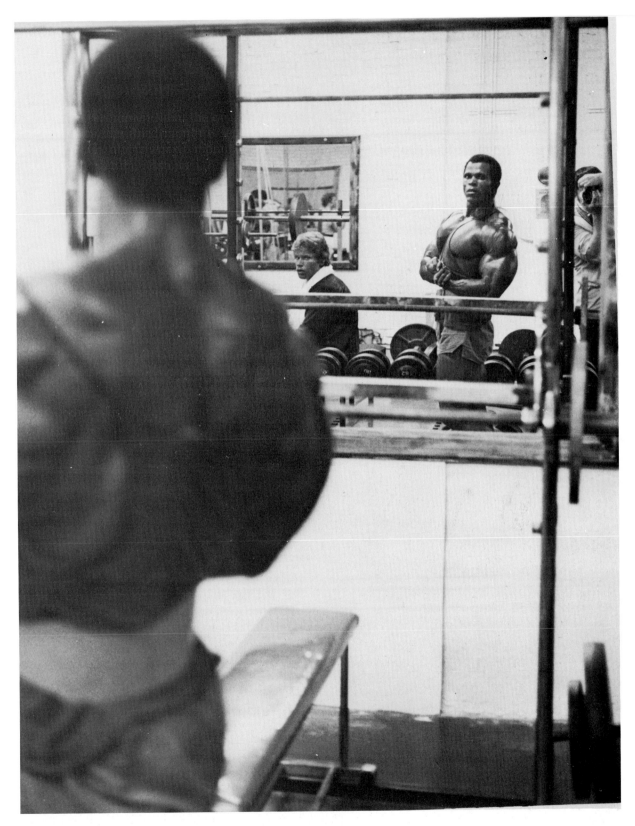

Practice posing with the help of a mirror whenever possible.

he was full of hot air. "You just weren't cut up enough, Arnold," retorted Joe between mouthfuls of filet steak.

Did Arnold ever concede that he was not in top shape that day in Miami when Zane trounced him? Yes. But it took him some twelve years. "Frank was better defined and tanned than I was," he finally coughed up. It took seven Olympia wins, innumerable successive victories over Zane, and twelve years' healing time before he had sufficient confidence to admit that maybe, just maybe, Frank had really deserved that title.

That is quite typical of bodybuilding egos. It would be very hard to find a champion who doesn't have this egocentric view of himself. Like the craft of acting, competitive bodybuilding demands that you "sell" yourself—one of the hardest things to do, especially on stage in front of a capacity audience. You simply cannot tell an actor that his acting is poor, and you can't tell a champion bodybuilder that he wasn't good enough to win.

If you suspect that *your* failure to win is due to "political" or other unfair reasons, then I urge you to consider that you may be wrong.

There are, of course, poor decisions in bodybuilding. I have witnessed many occasions when the wrong man won. But in the hundreds of contests I have witnessed, I have to say that for the most part the judges were genuinely sweating over making the right decision, and in the great majority of them the right man won.

Winning a contest is a matter of getting everything in line on the day of the competition. Size alone will never win a show, nor even size and definition, nor size and definition and proportion.

No sir, everything has to be right. Posing trunks must be well fitting. The cut of the thigh should be high, and the color should blend, harmonize, or contrast effectively with the tone of your skin. Striped, banded, or multicolored patterned trunks are out. The judges are scoring you, not your pose trunks. You should keep them simple, so that they don't distract attention from your physique. The best trunks, in my opinion, are those sold and advertised by Chris Dickerson and Frank Zane.

As pointed out earlier in this book, you've got to look tanned. You should endeavor to get the best natural tan possible, but even then, a few layers of Tan in a Minute, or Sudden Tan, or some other instant-tan concoction applied the last two days before a contest will help. Put on at least five layers (an hour apart). Very few natural tans are totally adequate, in that some areas (under the arms?) are less tanned than others.

Most black men need to sunbathe. There are a few who are so heavily pigmented that they could be considered *too* dark in the sense that the muscles do not show up fully, but there are very few like this. Among those whom I have seen too light and undertanned are Sergio Oliva, Chris Dickerson, Rick Wayne, Serge Nubret, Mohamed Makkawy, all men who have naturally dark skin, yet who have looked washed out and pale under the strong posing lights of a contest. Now each of them sunbathes before a show and looks a million percent better.

I have known Egyptians, Puerto Ricans, Lebanese, Indians, even dark-skinned Italians, all competing without a heavy tan. They felt they were dark enough. An Olympia contest will never be won by a man who is not sporting a maximum tan.

There have been many references to the use of creams and oils during a contest. Arnold Schwarzenegger used to rub in Nivea cream two or three times and then replace his sweatsuit and pump up. The resulting mixture of oil and sweat made his body glow with health on the posing plinth. Serge Nubret is another believer in creams. In fact, he never misses a day without coating his entire body with Nivea cream.

Today only a few bodybuilders use creams. The winners use oil (Johnson's Baby Oil) and nothing else.

Never completely relax on stage, even in the "relaxed" round. All eyes are on you, looking for flaws, so maintain an easy stride and a good posture. Hold your head high, and try not to keep staring down at your pecs or abs while on stage. Remember that charisma (the sparkling, confident personality that gives you power over the audience) is very important today—almost as important as muscles. It can certainly make the difference between winning and losing. Writer Jack Neary put it well: "Charisma is an elusive characteristic which few bodybuilders possess, but spectators easily recognize. It is fodder for a thousand essays, a progeny of confidence that is the bodybuilder's best friend when the sets are behind and the battle is at hand."

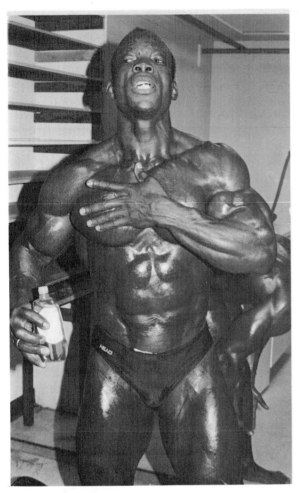
Oiling up: Al Beckles.

Make your poses dramatic, but not melo-dramatic. Good movement between poses is essential, but if it becomes superfluous, exaggerated, or affected, then it is no good.

During the last month of preparing for a contest, practice your posing for two half-hour periods each day. The last week you should pose for two one-hour periods daily, and this includes "crunching" the pecs and flexing muscles in all positions, not just in accepted poses. Practice keeping your thighs tensed for long periods. You will need this for the pre-judging part of the show, because even when you are not being directly appraised, the judges will still be looking your way now and again.

It will also help to practice holding your poses for long periods (30–60 seconds). Compulsory poses can be distinctly improved by practice.

A week before the show, get a haircut and shave your body. Then shave your body again the night before the show.

If the contest is on a Saturday, your last pre-contest workout should be on Wednesday night or Thursday morning. The two or three days of rest will let you recuperate enough to be at your best at the contest. Do nothing else but pose during these last days. No posing the morning of the show.

On the Friday night you may break your diet by having half a baked potato with your usual supper. On the Saturday you may have some scrambled egg with half a baked potato. During the morning, have an occasional slice of banana or apple to keep your glycogen level high for pumping. Even if you choose not to pump, your muscles will look fuller. Restrict your liquid intake to sips of water, but only when absolutely necessary.

Sergio Oliva in his heyday would have a virtually complete workout to pump his body prior to competing. Today, much less pumping is done. Basically, stretching movements like wide-grip chins are performed, together with dips and curls for chest and arms. Overpumped muscles take on a bloat. Definition and separation are lessened when your muscles are gorged with blood. Some pumping is good, though. You feel stronger, bigger, and you are more alert mentally.

Today's top bodybuilders will do anything to "stand out" on stage. Witness the fact that Mohamed Makkawy made his stage entrance at one New York Grand Prix . . . on a camel! Ken Passariello made his face up like the Kiss group and entered under the name of Demon.

It is my opinion that posing will become more dramatic during the next few years. That is to say, grace, poise, and even dance will be exhibited by some bodybuilders during their free posing. I also think there will be a return to *muscle control*, as practiced by men of the past like Maxalding and Stan Baker of England, and Ed Jubinville, Bruce Randall, and John Grimek of the USA. To get the jump on this coming trend, I suggest you practice muscle control techniques so that one day you will be able to wow an audience (and hopefully the judges) and bring home a first place trophy.

When not posing during the last few days before an important show, endeavor to rest a lot, and get your feet up. When you arrive at the auditorium, you will invariably have to wait before pumping up. Hanging around can be a drain on your nervous and physical energy. Try to lie down somewhere, and do your best to relax. It takes the edema (bloat) out of the body, and that will be one more feather in your cap, one that other competitors may not have thought of.

The last month's training before a contest is the most important of all. There is a fine line that you simply must travel. You should try and keep your exercise intensity high while limiting your food intake—no mean feat in itself. The intensity factor (not necessarily more sets, but more effort with heavy weights) will help to keep your size. But fewer calories will mean less energy, and possibly slower recuperation. This can lead to overwork. If you find yourself shaking excessively (trembling hands) during these pre-contest workouts, you may be delving too deeply into reserve energy. This will not only stop progress but will, in all likelihood, give your muscles a stringy, flat look. Even separation and

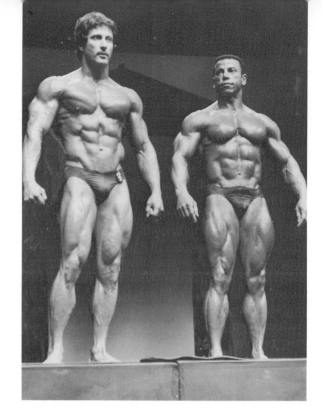

Both Frank Zane and Chris Dickerson, seen here at the 1982 Olympia in London, England, have that winner's look.

definition can suffer when the depleted nerve reservoirs fight to normalize the body's condition. Do *not* perform long workouts during your last four weeks of pre-contest training.

Bodybuilding is a thinking man's sport, regardless of what the general public might feel. You need to pay meticulous attention to *every* detail. You have to plan, experiment, evaluate, study, and analyze. My advice to you should be no more than food for thought. I do not know all the answers. You should listen not only to my advice but also to that of others with experience.

Experienced men are not all title winners. The greatest experts are often those who never had even an 18-inch arm. Among the most knowledgeable men in the field I would name Ken Wheeler, Bill Reynolds, Leo Stern, Jack Neary, Arthur Jones, John Balik, Norm Zale, Peary Rader, Denie, Clarence Bass, Vince Gironda—not the biggest men in the world, but they know their bodybuilding! There are, of course, knowledgeable top bodybuilders—Coe, Zane, Mentzer, Scott, Pearl—but a 20-inch arm is not necessarily the badge of bodybuilding expertise.

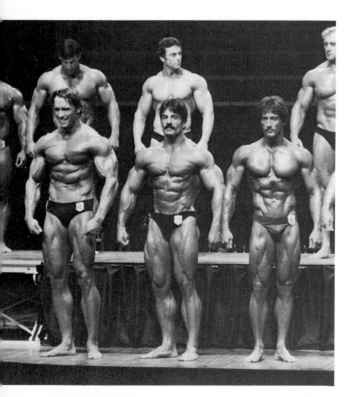

Practice standing in the "relaxed" position. You may have to do this for up to twenty minutes at a time in major contests.

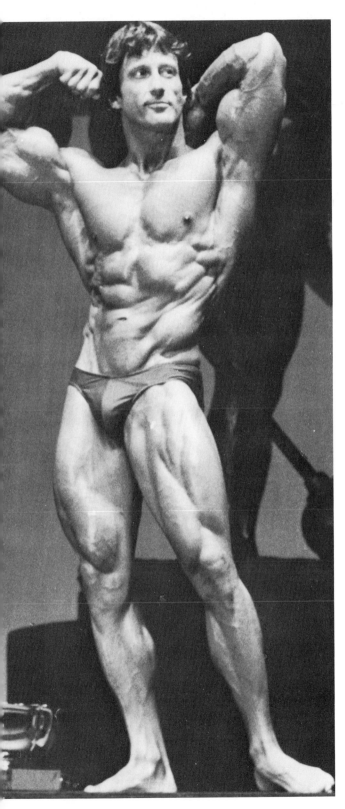
Zane—The master poser.

27

POSING
The Art
of
Successful
Physique
Display

What a man that "Buster" McShane was! I suppose one could say that he was larger than life. Certainly, his enthusiasm was larger than life and he had it in oodles.

Buster was an Irishman, full of humor and zest. He was a multiple Mr. Ireland winner and an oft-time training partner of Reg Park, who rocked the world of muscles in the 50's and 60's.

Hardly had I left my native England in 1968 and settled in Canada, but that Buster McShane paid me a visit. At the time I was a teacher at a local high school, and Buster delighted all the students by giving a weight-training demonstration free of charge. We had plenty of fun—training, drinking beer, and generally having a good time. Buster got a particular kick out of driving my new Jaguar all over the Canadian countryside. After he left, my bench press quickly dropped the 30 pounds it had risen during his stay.

Buster was killed a few years later in Ireland, while driving home from a party in his new Jaguar V-12. Apparently, he had fallen asleep at the wheel and driven into a brick wall. Death was instantaneous. Those damn Jag's always ran hot! Many a time I got drowsy on a long night's drive.

When I think of Buster McShane I always smile because he once had me rolling around laughing so much I thought I would split my sides. We had just stepped into an elevator on our way to the top of a big Toronto hotel. When the elevator doors closed, the music was automatically piped in. Lo and behold, it was "Legend of the Glass Mountain," Buster's favorite posing music! Without hesitation, he dropped to his knees and lost himself to the music, posing with heart and soul and complete abandon. Buster was drawing his routine to a close with a red-faced, all-out "most muscular," when the elevator doors parted and revealed him to an audience of a dozen people. As we rolled out of the elevator convulsed with loud laughter, they gave us some pretty funny looks.

Posing is everything in bodybuilding competitions. It shows you at your best and at your worst. Charles Gaines, of *Pumping Iron* fame, said it perfectly: "Posing is the art of the thing. Depending on how it is done, you can see in it either everything that is moving and beautiful and dignified about the display of a developed body, or everything that is ridiculous and embarrassing about it."

The way you pose at a contest is the sum total of your endeavors. It's your showpiece. Perfection is never achieved, but you can reach out to grasp as much of it as humanly possible.

The first thing you should understand is that in today's contests a bodybuilder is showing much more than his muscles, especially when it comes to professional competition. In addition to having large, balanced, well-defined and tanned muscles, our super-hero of the platform must exude confidence, have a feel for the music and for the shapes his body makes during and between poses, should possess an air of mystical excitement and a flair for the dramatic. All this should go with a decided penchant for communicating with the audience and with a charisma that exudes from his entire personality.

Music and timing go together, of course. Today's pro bodybuilder has to co-ordinate his posing to music. As a dyed-in-the-wool hardcore bodybuilder, you may find this idea offensive, but it is essential to ultimate success.

Many amateur contests do not allow competitors to choose their own music, so here the problem of choosing the right music doesn't exist. Nonetheless, the aspiring bodybuilder should practice posing to suitable music. It will help him in the long run; and even if he doesn't turn professional, he may be asked to guest-pose at shows or at other functions, and his routine will look all the more polished if he has practiced the performance to inspiring music.

The question of what type of music you should pose to cannot be answered authoritatively, because styles change. In the 60's, it was common for bodybuilders to pose to "Legend of the Glass Mountain." In fact, Reg Park wore out half a dozen records of this music, posing all over the world in the 50's and 60's. Subsequently, "Exodus" and some Wagner be-

Like a god from the sea: the one and only Arnold Schwarzenegger.

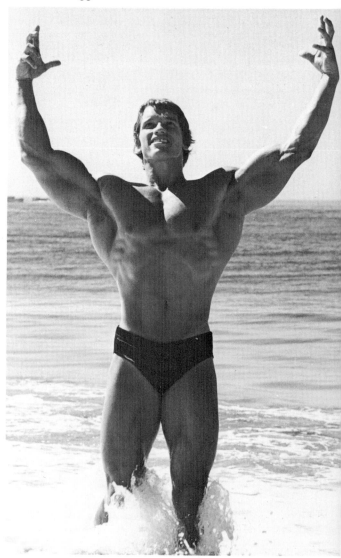

160

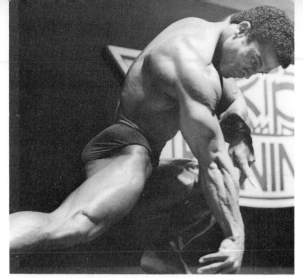
Mohamed Makkawy has superb posing skills.

came favorites, and then it was "Rocky" and "Eye of the Tiger."

Currently, many bodybuilders are posing to disco beat or hard-rock scores. Perhaps one day classical music will be in vogue, but at present it does not bring audience and poser together.

For sure, good music can help a bodybuilder win a contest. You must try to find the ideal piece for your routine. Bear in mind the points to look for: your posing music must be, at least partly, known to the audience; it should accent your poses; it must build to a peak; and it must draw the spectators into what you are doing on stage by touching either their emotions or their innate sense of rhythm.

I have seen a bodybuilder pose to a dull part of his music and get very little audience response, only to repeat the same poses to a more inspiring part of the tape and almost bring the audience to its feet. This is no exaggeration. Music has the power to make people cheer, dance, groan, or weep. In fact, it can motivate one to almost anything. Adolf Hitler roused a nation to accept his challenge, however misguided, by his power of oratory combined with classical German music.

Writing in *Muscle and Fitness*, musician David Lasker says that bodybuilders should use the musician's "trick" of counting during their posing: "Like a musician, you must count the beats in each bar of music. It will serve to pace your routine correctly."

Actually, learning to count is easy. Your posing music is divided into measures, or bars, of four (or three) beats each. Count them: one, two, three, four. You have counted one complete

bar, or measure. Some music, such as waltzes, has only three beats to a bar.

Lasker also suggests that you listen carefully for the strong and weak bars. A strong bar begins with a cymbal crash or a loud, accented chord. This is the moment to sweep in and *hit* a pose. During weak bars you may simply hold your poses or glide into another attitude. Consider the number of poses in a routine (10–20?), then choose a piece of music that has the right number of strong bars to accommodate and do justice to your own posing display.

Many professional bodybuilders try to map out a routine by counting the strong and weak bars and then memorize them in order to synchronize their poses with the chosen music. However, since little if any music was written with a bodybuilder's pose-routine in mind, very few pieces lend themselves completely to the bodybuilder's needs. So it is not uncommon for a pro bodybuilder to take his tape to a professional sound studio and have some of the music edited out in order to tailor the sounds to his needs. I can foresee the day when music will be especially written for individual pose routines.

More and more show promoters are allowing contestants to bring along their own tapes, so if you are at all serious about bodybuilding competition, then you must practice until you can go through your routine almost automatically. Do not leave anything to chance. If you rely on the inspiration of the moment, then chances are you will fail to make the impression you wanted to make.

Another original Makkawy pose.

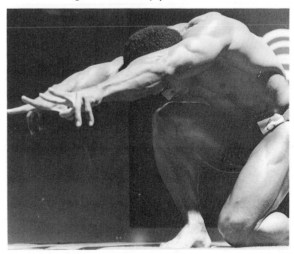

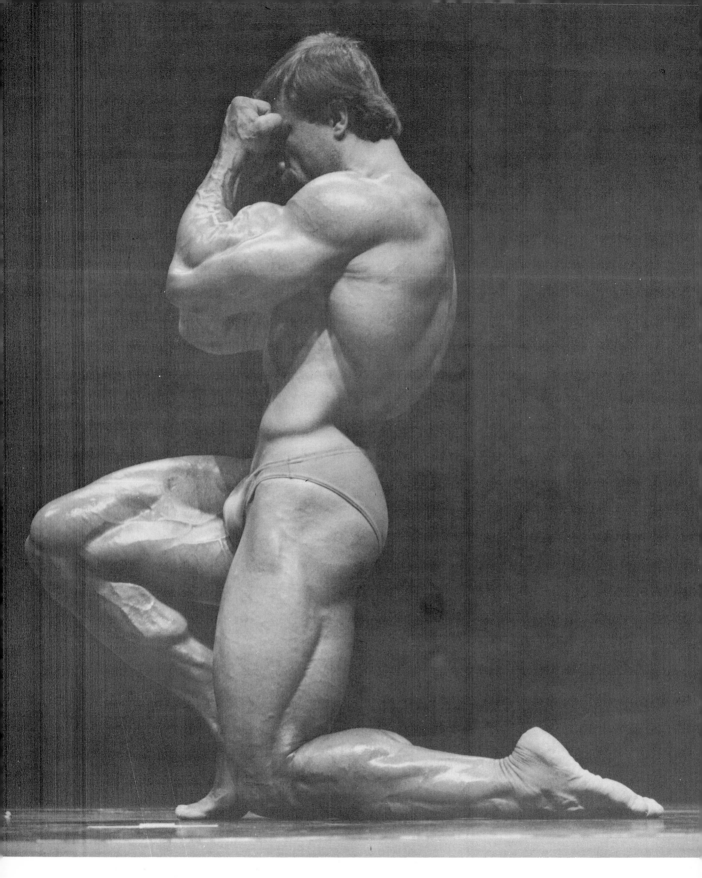

A beautiful pose—Ali Mala shows how.

Whenever you practice your posing, count the bars (pose No. 1 lasts X bars, pose No. 2 lasts Y bars). This will help you duplicate your routine exactly each time. It will also reduce on-stage "nerves," because you'll have something to occupy your mind.

Exactly what poses to perform is a totally individual thing. Each bodybuilder has poses which only he can do effectively. Could it be argued that Bertil Fox does not "own" the kneeling arms-straight-down pose, or that Arnold's three-quarter back shot has not been equalled?

One thing is for sure: you must practice your posing. Apart from the compulsory poses

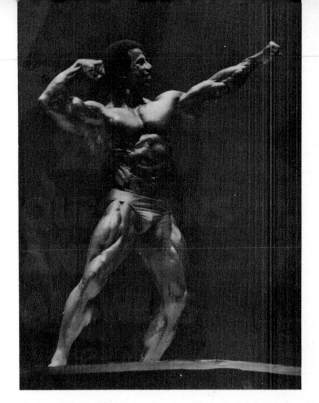

One of the all-time master posers: Chris Dickerson.

Winning the 1979 Mr. Olympia—Frank Zane.

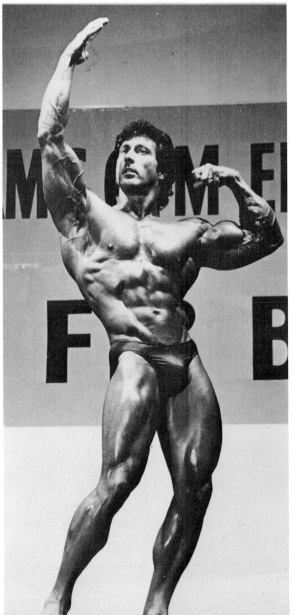

(side chest, front abdominal, front and back double biceps, lat spread from front and back), you must develop an arsenal of free poses to use during the free posing round. You will get most of your ideas by looking at the various books and magazines available. When you practice posing, use a full-length mirror, and adjust the light to show your muscles to their best advantage.

I strongly recommend that you never give up on a pose. In the case of the compulsory poses you simply *cannot* give up. They are your bread-and-butter point getters in competition.

Practice *all* poses. Even if a particular attitude does not suit you, practice it. Your body will grow into it. Obviously, when you perform for a judging panel you will include only your best poses, but you should still practice a large variety of poses. The flexing, stretching, and twisting will help you look better, and it will complement the work you have done in the gym. If you find the art of posing particularly difficult, then by all means seek help from professionals who know about movement and stage presence. Ballet schools may be able to help. But before you enroll in a ballet class, make sure it is understood just what you are trying to accomplish. It is not your intention to perform "Swan Lake" in ballet tights!

163

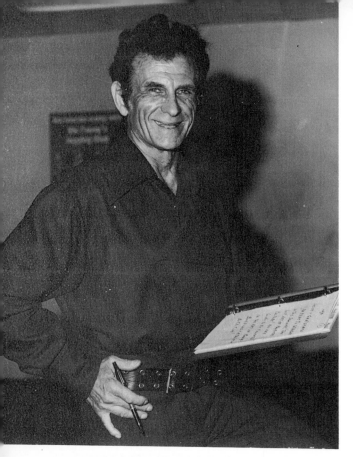

Vince Gironda. The champs go to him for posing and training advice.

Granted it's not easy to turn on to a bunch of judges, or an audience, at least not as effectively as you do in front of your own bathroom mirror, but constant practice will make it easier and easier each successive time.

Although you can refer to books and magazines for individual poses, you will have to see live bodybuilders (if only on film or tape) to learn the secrets of how to move between poses. The entire routine must be studied. It is a good idea to try and see a professional show, especially something as prestigious as the IFBB Mr. Olympia. Even so, some competitors will be far superior to others. Among the all-time great posers are Sig Klein, John Grimek, Clancy Ross, Reg Park, Frank Zane, Ed Corney, Chris Dickerson, and Mohamed Makkawy.

From amateur contests, except at the national and international level, you can seldom learn how to pose. Typically, each contestant starts with a double biceps and ends with a distorted, arm-flapping (to bring out the vascularity) "most muscular." In between we are treated to an assortment of shuffles, groans, and grunts, accompanied by awkward attempts to flex up under duress. Occasionally, though, you will witness a posing phenomenon at an amateur show. He may not be the best built, and he may not even place in the contest, but his routine will be one of the most memorably magnificent. Watch and learn from these rarities.

Bear in mind that styles change. There are no rules "carved in stone" for the present-day poser. One could glibly suggest that a routine should incorporate drama, changes of pace and rhythm, smiles and charisma. Yet who's to say that the next master poser to come along will utilize these features? If we could drop in on Eugene Sandow's first physique contest at London's Royal Albert Hall some eighty years ago, we would no doubt be bored to tears. Far from clapping our hands in enthusiastic applause, we would probably use them to stifle a draggle of yawns. Looking eighty years into the future, it is just as likely that our descendants will be yawning at what we now consider a gut-bustin' display of muscle and might.

When you practice your routine in front of your bathroom mirror, try closing your eyes before you hit each pose. After you have "fixed" your position, open your eyes and check out the result.

Always aim to look confident as you pose. A smile will beat out a frown any day. You are only kidding yourself if you think that all you need is muscles to come out on top in a bodybuilding contest.

Kozo Sudo, the Japanese champion.

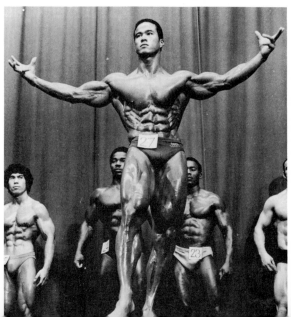

It is important that you only use poses that highlight your physique. Copying someone else's routine pose-for-pose is totally impractical. Each of us is different, and by virtue of that fact, your posing routine must be unique.

Basically, if you are lacking in size, you shouldn't spread out your legs or arms in your poses. Always remember that if you *do* stretch out, to do so proudly. Nothing looks worse than a pointing arm that isn't straight, because the poser feels insecure about fully stretching out. Be proud: go to the extreme, straighten out to the limit. Have nothing, absolutely nothing, to be ashamed of, because you can bet your last dollar it will be communicated to the audience.

Never try to egg on the audience to applaud. They may respond, but will really resent your action. An audience doesn't pay money to be told what to do by a performer.

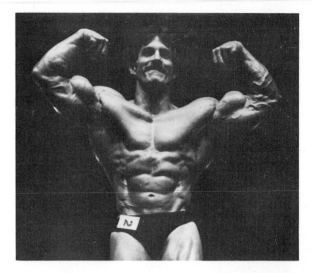

An unbelievable double biceps—Mike Mentzer.

When you pose, your movements are being watched by every eye in the auditorium. A smile will let the people know that your mind is communicating with them as you go through your routine. When you are a good poser you will have the audience enthralled. Your movements will command attention. The crowd will be eating out of your hands. Unlike the work of exercising for muscles, where overtraining will lead to staleness, the constant practice of posing, especially the performance of a complete routine, will only serve to fine-tune your presentation and to improve your competitiveness. Master the art of physique display, and you are a winner. Fail to master it, and your chance of success is greatly diminished.

Al Beckles of Britain.

Makkawy has everything together.

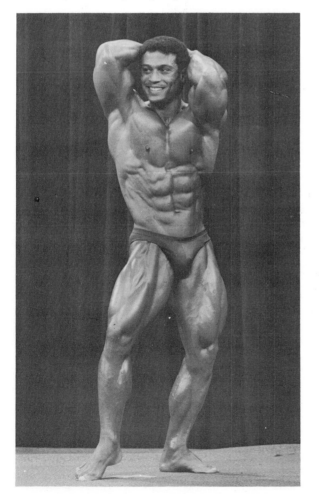

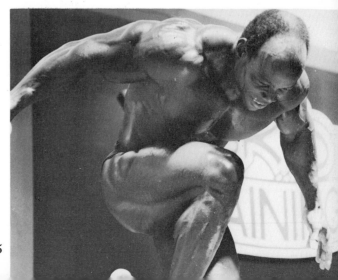

Master poser Chris Dickerson
shows how his magnificent
routine transpires . . .

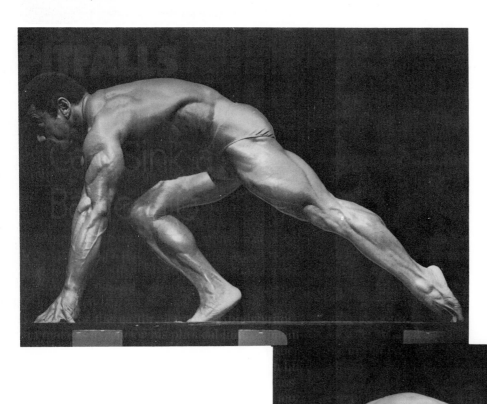

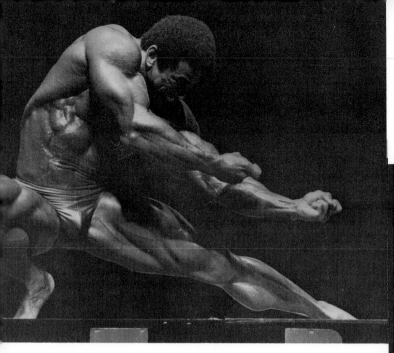

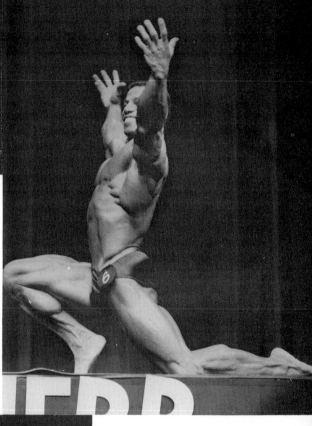

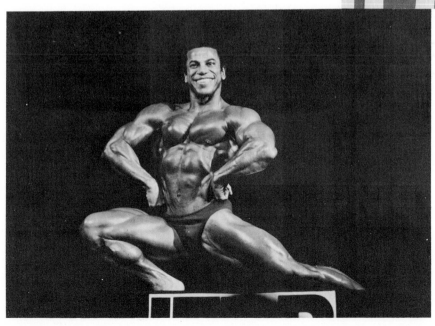

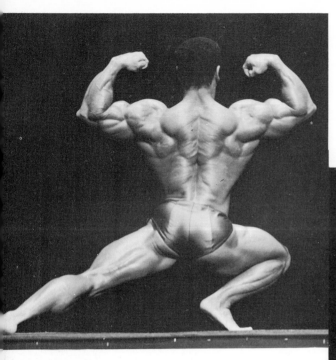

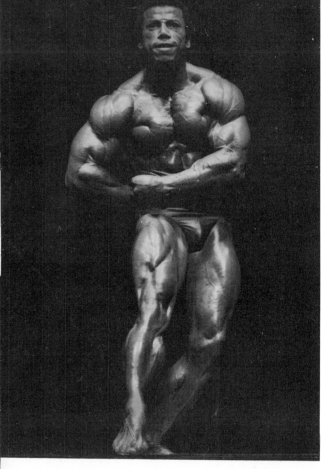

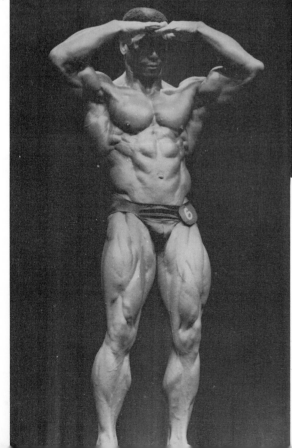

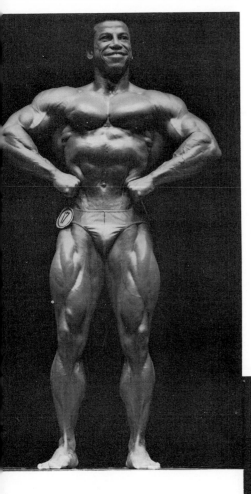

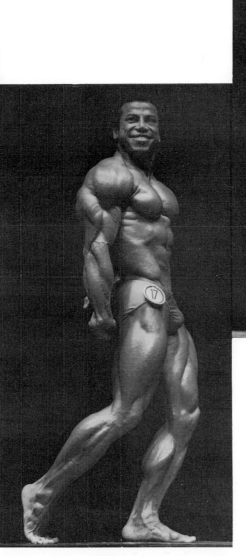

28

THE TEN BODYBUILDING PITFALLS

Small Leaks Can Sink a Battleship

One of the cardinal errors a bodybuilder can make is to rely for his physical improvement entirely on a routine of weight training or other progressive resistance exercises. "If only I can hit on the ideal training program," he thinks, "muscular magnificence would be mine within a few months!" This is just not true. Some routines will undoubtedly be more effective than others, but there is no *one* schedule that will bring sensational, unending gains. And like any other endeavor, bodybuilding has its pitfalls, and you must attempt to avoid them at all costs.

Overtraining

It is very difficult to overwork the muscles of a trained athlete, but very easy indeed to drive the nervous system too hard. Clinical and laboratory experiments indicate that the muscles themselves can withstand phenomenal demands. But when a bodybuilder continues an exercise until he cannot perform another repetition, he runs the risk (especially if this is done for a prolonged period) of causing an injury, or at least a breakdown. It is the nervous system

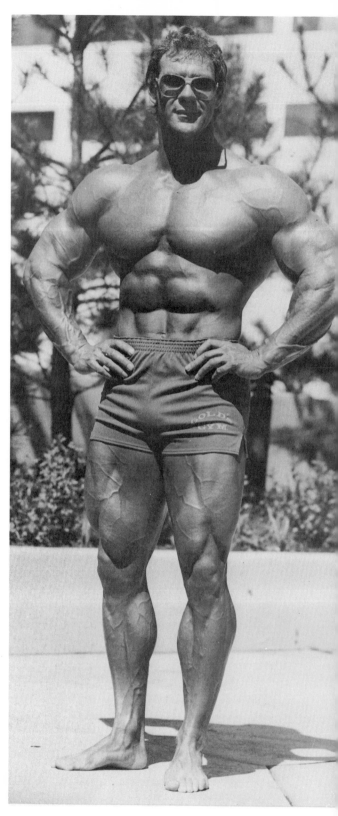

Scott Wilson. He pays attention to every aspect of bodybuilding. No pitfalls.

rather than the muscle fibre which is unable to cope. According to physiologists, the first to fatigue in the neuro-muscular system are the motor cells in the brain; next come the nerve "end-plates"; and in the third place, the muscle fibres themselves. The nerve itself is almost unfatiguable. As a result of repeated consecutive muscular contractions, chemical changes occur at the nerve endings which make the transmission of the nerve impulse increasingly difficult, so that the brain has to provide a stronger stimulus via its motor cells to keep the repetitions going.

Forcing oneself in an exercise on a regular or prolonged basis past reasonable fatigue to exhaustion is therefore very expensive in nervous energy and can, according to Dr. Clifford Amenduri, shut your insulin production down. It is quite evident that the best bodybuilding gains are made by those who either limit their all-out training to infrequent intervals or drive themselves just far enough, but not too far.

Undernourishment

Are you, especially if you are a young beginning bodybuilder, getting adequate food for your muscle to grow? Often youngsters are walking "power stations." With their high metabolisms, they burn up fuel at an unbelievable rate. To make matters worse, many of these fellows actually miss breakfast. How can you expect to have sufficient energy to supply your ordinary needs and have enough fuel also for adding solid muscle to your frame?

I am against pigging out or force-feeding the body to bring about bodyweight gains, but you can't create something out of nothing. Maybe Rome wasn't built in a day, but let's face it, Rome would not have been built in even a trillion years without the bricks to do the job. Check over the nutrition chapter in this book and make sure you are feeding your muscles sufficiently for that all-important growth you want to achieve.

Nutritional Overloading

In its way, eating too much is as bad as not eating enough, and it is just as common. The unfortunate result is that for every inch you gain on your chest you add two inches on your waist.

A trip to fat-city seldom reverses itself. At least not without enormous dedication and perseverance. Once fat is comfortably sitting around your tummy, your lower back, and your hips, it is not easily dislodged. Like a dog that is chased from a comfortable bed, it will return at the slightest opportunity, and often when you are not aware of it.

Fat kills your appearance. Ironically, a covering of "lard" will make you look bigger in clothes (even though your pudgy face will give out your true condition), but when stripped at the beach, pool, or lake, you will look smaller than if you carried almost pure muscle.

The things that make a shaped up, muscular bodybuilder look good are the curves of his muscles—the way the delts run into the arms, the "peak" of the biceps, the delineation of the three heads of the triceps, the separation of the quadriceps, not to mention the absence of fat around the knee, ankle, and elbow joints. All these eye-catching phenomena are lost if there is a preponderance of fat. Superfluous weight fills in the crevices between the muscles which would add to their dramatic appearance.

When your waist–chest differential diminishes instead of increasing, you know you are in trouble. Cut the calories before it is too late. You've become a resident of fat-city without even knowing it. Get out of town quick!

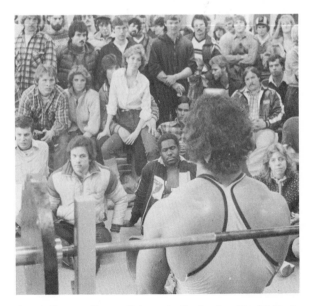

A captive audience listens to Barbarian David Paul as he explains bodybuilding and its problems.

Faulty Proportion

Nothing inspires like success when the bodybuilder notices that his chest or thighs, or what have you, is growing. So what does he do? Why, he works that growing area even more—like you wouldn't believe! He doubles his sets of squats, and triples his bench presses. Whatever area grows best, he will work on twice as hard as before. "As if increase of appetite grew by what it fed on," said Hamlet.

This, of course, leads to the demon *disproportion*. The guy may have no arms or calves, or a lousy back, but his pecs and thighs are growing like crazy. They go beyond good, all the way to superb, but in the wake of their progress, the lagging body parts look and become progressively worse.

Training for proportion is a little tricky because some parts grow faster than others. The slower-growing parts probably have a lesser allocation of muscle cells. Slow-growth areas must not be worked with as many sets or with similar intensity as the faster growing groups—they must be worked with *more*!

Injury from Poor Exercise Form

Avoid injury by *never* randomly attempting a near-limit weight. Two years ago I jokingly said to a friend of mine, Gino Edwards, "See that dumbbell? In the old days when we were kids we would jerk press that overhead easily with one hand." Within a few seconds Gino had taken my casual remarks to heart and had hoisted the weight (a 150-pound dumbbell) overhead. He put it up at arm's length and lowered it with a smile. As he stood upright, the smile evaporated. He clasped his trapezius, grunted, groaned, and cursed. His subsequent pinched-nerve condition has taken one and a-half inches of development from his left arm and lessened his strength by 50 percent. Needless to say, even today, two years later, he has not fully recovered. I am no longer in his good books.

Injury usually occurs from showing off, from attempting a new limit, or from sloppy exercise form. The most easily injured area appears to be the complex shoulder pectoral area, but any muscle can sustain a tear, strain, or other injury. Warm up adequately and use proper exercise style. If you bounce the weight up when doing scott preacher curls, or jerk the barbell when rowing, or "drop" into heavy full squats, then injury will visit you with a vengeance one day.

Neglecting Aerobic Exercise

Many bodybuilders feel that aerobic exercise (prolonged exercise that works the heart and lungs steadily and increases cardiovascular fitness) is a waste of time. During a specific bulk or weight gain period you may choose not to perform any type of exercise other than your heavy gym training, but aerobic exercise does have the following advantages:
1. It helps to keep your fat level down.
2. It improves your wind during tough exercises like squats and so prevents your lungs from giving out before your legs.
3. It aids recuperation and inspires regularity of appetite and bowels.
4. It hypes the metabolism.

On the last rep, Dennis Tinerino goes all out. Expert training knowledge keeps him ahead.

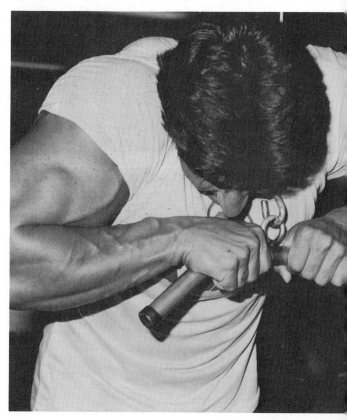

172

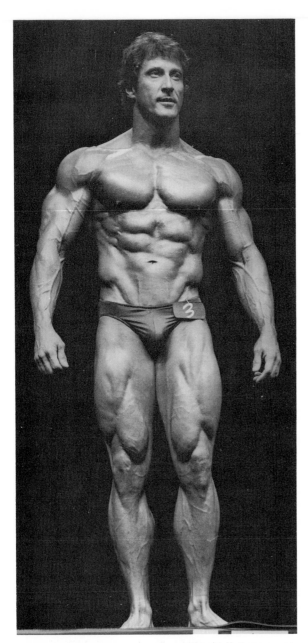

Perfect proportion is the trademark of three-time IFBB Olympia winner Frank Zane.

Smoking and Drinking

Both are bad in excess. Drink is tolerable in moderation, smoking is not.

I have known many bodybuilders who smoked. Although some had their trophy winning days, none lasted the course.

The simple fact is that a bodybuilder needs an abundance of energy and pep. Cigarette smoking takes away both. The first thing to suffer is the squat. The cigarette smoker just can't do the reps. Soon his workouts deteriorate to becoming a joke, and ultimately the physique mirrors the low-quality training. For the cigarette smoker, his days of hope for success are numbered.

Drink, in moderation, especially with meals is acceptable, but cannot be continued during specific contest preparation. Arnold Schwarzenegger always liked a glass or two of wine or champagne, but when he was preparing for a contest, not a drop passed his lips.

If you like to down a bottle of whisky or fill your stomach to the limit with beer over the weekend, then you are overindulging. Your drinking has got the better of you, and success will elude you as far as contest-winning bodybuilding is concerned. Moderation is the key.

Extra Exercise

Do not bemoan your inability to gain weight if you in any way resemble the proverbial human dynamo who fritters away his energy in a weekly routine of soccer, bowling, two evenings of racquet-ball, three evenings of roller-skating, and a weekend of disco dancing. By all means enjoy occasional friendly games and pas-

Ulf Benggsten of Sweden.

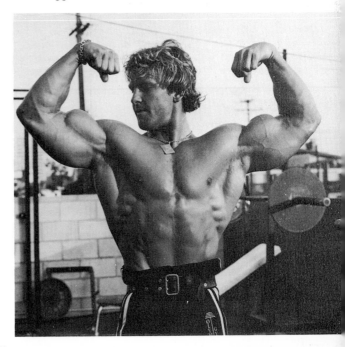

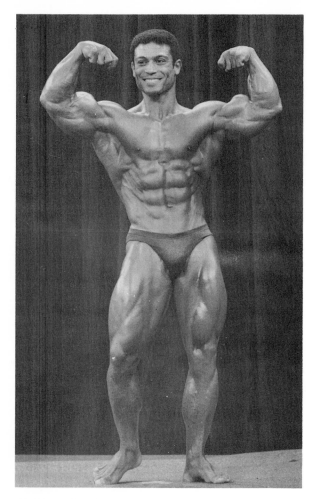
Mohamed Makkawy has one of the most complete physiques in the world.

the "most muscular." Anything else makes them look "bunched-up."

I must admit that I am against the use of artificial steroids, but even if I had no second thoughts about their safety, I would still regard them as the enemy of the young bodybuilder. They don't make him look any better. For one thing, they tend to bloat and thicken the waistline.

Other drugs that bodybuilders use—from diuretics to thyroid—all cause physical damage of one kind or another, and those who rely on them for muscle and shape never come out on top in the end.

Dr. Lynne Pirie, a competitive bodybuilder in her own right, says: "Diuretics cause electrolyte imbalance, which can cause damage and precipitate arrhythmia, an abnormality of the cardiac rhythm."

As a bodybuilder you may feel invincible, but if you neglect your health, you will quickly find out that you are not.

Listening to So-called Friends

Sometimes enemies can be more helpful to a bodybuilder than friends. How come? In order to put you down, an enemy may point out all your physical faults, while a friend, or one who pretends to be, will tell you what you want to hear rather than the truth. Many a time I have seen "friends" telling competing bodybuilders that "they wuz robbed," when in reality they were lucky to place where they did. It is hard for a bodybuilder to see how he looks up on stage in the company of other competitive bodybuilders, so he relies on the opinion of others. The opinion they voice is often not really their true opinion but merely a valentine to allay the performer's unhappiness.

I am not suggesting that you should adopt a negative attitude towards yourself, but nothing is worse than acting as though you should have won a contest when the whole audience knows differently. In one show I attended, two competitors who failed to place in the Top 3, threw their 5th and 6th place trophies at the judges in the front row of the audience. On that occasion, the winner was deservedly in first place, and those two aggressive maniacs were lucky, in my opinion, to have done as well as they did.

times, but at a time when you are trying to add muscle to your bony frame, keep other physical activities in perspective. Be prepared to abandon other physically demanding pursuits until you have obtained and consolidated your required muscular gains.

Relying on Steroids and Other Drugs

Anabolic steroids are not a substitute for hard work. They will increase the liquid retention of your muscles, which will make them bigger in appearance. The buffer effect will also allow you to lift heavier weights, but too many youngsters use steroids instead of really tough training. They are often in poor physical condition. The only pose they can effectively present is

Lou Ferrigno, one of the most famous bodybuilders of all. He is the training inspiration of half the world.

29

QUESTIONS AND ANSWERS
Help!

Lateral Triceps

Question: I want to develop the lateral (outer) head of my triceps. I greatly admire this area of the arm, but only a handful of bodybuilders seem to have exceptional development in this region. Steve Reeves had it, and I see really great lateral triceps on Dennis Tinerino and Mohamed Makkawy also. How can I get this impressiveness?

Answer: When fully developed, the lateral head of the tricep does add drama and quality to upper arm appearance. In fact, the entire arm benefits. Most two-handed triceps exercises in which the hands are closer together than the elbows work the outer head vigorously. Makkawy uses the kneeling overhead pulley press, while Tinerino also uses the close-grip bench press with EZ curl bar and the triceps lat-machine pressdowns with the elbows held out to the sides.

Steve Reeves found that the single-arm lying dumbbell stretch effected great stress on the lateral triceps head. The dumbbell (start with a light weight because perfect style is essential) is lowered *across* the chest, so that when the right arm is exercised, the dumbbell is lowered to the left pectoral.

175

How Much Muscle?

Question: I have just begun bodybuilding. How much muscle can I expect to gain in the first year? How do I know what potential I have?

Answer: No one can say for sure, and it is too hard to assess your potential accurately by measuring, weighing, or looking at you. Many champions were skinny to begin with. Beginners often gain quickly. If you eat well, train progressively on a regular basis, and sleep well, you will be on the right track for gaining 10, 15, or 20 pounds during your first year. Beyond this, body weight can be gained by forced feeding, but a great deal of what you gain will be fat. Intermediate bodybuilders seldom gain more than 7 or 8 pounds of pure muscle a year, often considerably less.

Charlie Thomas of New York.

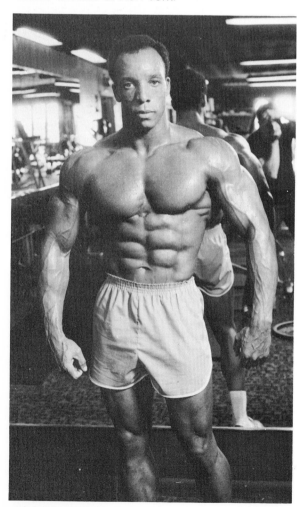

Cellulite

Question: I have been exercising with weights as well as stretching and running for more years than I can recall, but lately I have noticed a dimpled effect on my backside. I need your advice on how to rid myself of this unsightly appearance.

Answer: What you have on your seat is *fat!* It has become fashionable to refer to this dimpled effect as "cellulite," but in fact it is simply fat. It tends to be stored in large amounts on the upper thighs and bottom and tends to dimple the skin surface because it is pulled downwards by gravity.

The beauty industry has come up with numerous so-called cellulite cures—like creams and gels to massage in, pills to break up fat and prevent fluid retention, heat treatments to draw out toxic body waters, and injections of "anti-cellulite" serums. However, though some of these methods may prove marginally successful, by far the best way to rid yourself of this fat is to redesign your diet so that your overall calorie count is lowered. In addition, you may want to increase the speed and severity of your workouts so that more calories are burned. By attacking the problem on two fronts, success is that much more likely. You will not easily work off the dimpled fat effect without reorganizing your diet.

Bigger Wrists

Question: I have just read my first bodybuilding magazine, so I am writing you with this question: How can I enlarge the size of my wrists?

Answer: Wrist size increases naturally up to somewhere in your mid-twenties. All weight trainers, especially those who train with heavy weights, gain some wrist size, due to actual bone growth (thickness) and to the sinews and tendons that surround the wrist. There is no specific growing exercise for the wrist.

What Are They Doing?

Question: Whenever I look at a bodybuilding magazine I am shocked at the fantastic "ripped-up" look of the muscles on the various bodybuilders. How do these men do it? I train extremely hard, eat well, take protein supplements, and have developed some pretty good muscles, but can't even imagine myself ever looking as defined and trained as those men in the magazines. How is it they look like this all the time? I mean what are they doing that I don't do? I have become pretty dejected because I just don't seem to measure up to these human anatomy charts. I would like an answer as soon as possible please.

Answer: You have made the incorrect assumption that many have made before you. The top bodybuilding champs are not always in super-ripped shape. In fact, often their super muscularity is only evident for a few days before and after a contest. Like every other sportsman (yes, every sportsman), the bodybuilder must hit his peak right on the day of competition. When the peak is reached there is a natural (and needed) period of relaxation. This is very evident in sports like boxing and our event, bodybuilding.

In their ordinary training, most bodybuilders coast along trying to specialize on improving a lagging body part in order to increase overall proportions, or working with heavier and heavier weights to add size and strength. But once a contest is in sight, their methodology changes. They must, among other things, think of reaching their best contest weight right at the time of competition. The pictures you see in the magazines are nearly always taken within a few days of an important competition. Many, of course, are taken on the day of competition, either while posing on stage or else under studio lights set up backstage. So do remember that when you see top bodybuilders "ripped to shreds" in the various magazines, they are not like this all the time.

I think it only fair to tell you that many bodybuilders peaking for a contest resort to potentially dangerous drugs, like thyroid or excessive diuretics, coupled with near-starvation diets. Accordingly, on the day of the show they are prone to cramps, nervousness, and even heart irregularities which can cause lasting health problems and may shorten their career as well as their life span.

After the peak has been reached, there is a natural and necessary period of relaxation. Some champion bodybuilders actually give up all training after a contest and follow some other interest or activity. Steve Reeves frequently did this when he felt a need to devote more time to

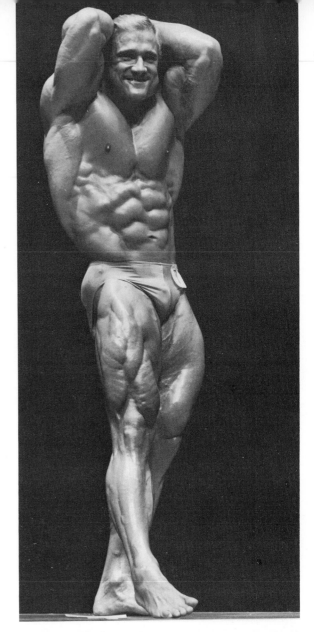

Tom Platz. Ready and ripped!

his acting. Frank Zane loves archery. Arnold enjoys scuba diving, distance running, and skiing. Serge Nubret takes the entire winter off. Most bodybuilders, however, because they love training, actually work out all year round, especially the "hungry" amateurs who want to get to the top in a hurry. As a hard-training bodybuilder you have a choice of either looking big and beefy all year round, or looking slightly smaller but muscularly impressive. What you cannot be is big and super-ripped all year. That is possible only at the conclusion of a planned peaking operation, which needs tremendous motivation, a restricted diet, and intensive training.

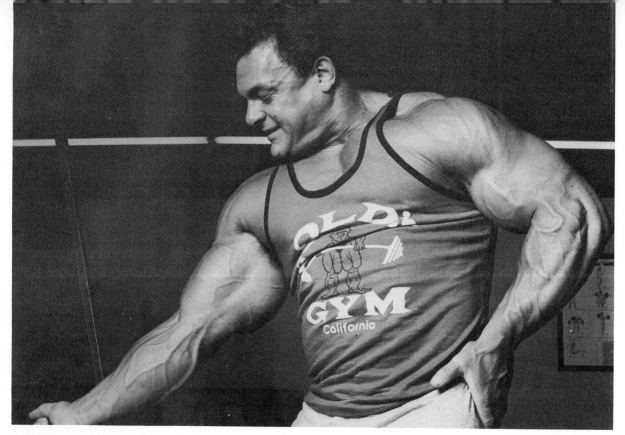

Tim Belknap, Mr. America.

Heart Attack

Question: I am forty-seven years old and I am worried about having a heart attack some day soon. To be honest, I have smoked for thirty years. I always drink at least a quart of milk with breakfast (3 eggs and bacon). In addition, I have a high-stress job. The good news is that I have been working out with weights since I was a kid. What can I do to lessen my chances of having a heart attack? I have lost several friends to this disease.

Answer: You do not say whether you have been having chest pains or whether you have some foundation, like your heredity, for fearing a heart attack. If so, see your doctor for a proper checkup.

I would cut down on heavy fats, if I were you. Certainly stop smoking, since there is a direct relation between smoking and heart problems. Regular exercise is helpful to the heart, but it is no guarantee against heart disease. I strongly suggest you eat plenty of fruits rich in bioflavonoids, which serve to protect you from heart disease, strengthen capillaries, and help to prevent plugged up arteries. Your best fruits are oranges, lemons, tangerines, grapefruit, apples, pears, limes, plums, and cherries.

Awkward Bodybuilders

Question: I have observed that many top bodybuilding stars look awkward when standing normally. Some have poor shape and look unimpressive. In my opinion, only a few bodybuilders look good standing relaxed.

Answer: I agree with you, and so does the IFBB judging hierarchy. That is why we have a "relaxed" judging round, where the competitors are viewed from front, back, and sides in the normal position. The reason why so many top bodybuilders look unimpressive in the relaxed position is that steroids have allowed their muscles to overcrowd their frame. They look bunched up! Bodybuilders who look good just standing there often have wide shoulders and comparatively narrow hips. The choice example, of course, is Sergio Oliva. Other impressive men include Dennis Tinerino, Serge Nubret, Robbie Robinson, Danny Padilla, Frank Zane, and Mike Mentzer.

I Want Veins

Question: I want big veins in my chest, back, and legs. I will be entering a contest soon, and I need to develop extreme vascularity of the type that Clint Beyerle and Don Ross have. Should I take large doses of niacin and thyroid?

Answer: Definitely not! Taking thyroid can knock out your own thyroid gland, and high-dosage niacin can knock your eyeballs to the back of your head. Leave them alone!

Why on earth would you want maximum vascularity? Ugly, bulging crisscross veins usually run contrary to the lines of the muscle separation and totally detract from any shape or mass you might possess. Your thinking is extremely distorted. Veins don't make a physique, muscles do. A degree of vascularity is fine, but too much is the trademark of an amateur, not of a winner. If you had your way, the judges would be eyeballing your ugly veins and nothing else.

Headaches

Question: I have been getting a lot of headaches lately. They seem to come when I squat or do heavy pressing exercises. Often they go away when I finish my workout. Could my training be causing these headaches? I enjoy using forced reps and negatives and would hate to have to ease up on my training.

Answer: Sometimes training increases internal pressure, and this could cause your headaches, but there are a thousand and one causes of headaches. The room could be too hot; you may have high blood pressure; it could be the stress factor or excessive noise—the list is endless. I have no solution other than to say, I have had headaches from training, and so have many people with me. They have usually occurred when I went a bit crazier than usual with my training, especially after a layoff. Perhaps you are not quite ready for forced reps yet. I suggest you reduce the intensity and length of your training for a while and attempt to build up slowly again. If the headaches persist, see your doctor.

Forearms Blow Up

Question: I hope you can help me with a problem I have had since Day 1 of my training.

Whenever I do biceps and triceps work, especially biceps, my forearms blow up like crazy. The pump hurts so much, I have to stop a set before my upper arms are fully worked. My forearms are 15½ and my upper arms are only 16½ fully flexed. I feel and look like Popeye. Please tell me which upper arm movements I can do so that my forearms won't blow up each set.

Answer: Men like Mike Mentzer have this same problem, and in one sense you can consider yourself fortunate. You may never have to do specialized forearm work because your forearms will always receive adequate stimulation from regular upper arm exercises. Many bodybuilders have to do 10–12 sets of forearm movements just to keep their lower arms "in line" with their upper arms.

Your particular muscle cell allocation and leverage makeup will dictate which exercises you can do without getting congested forearms. You will have to experiment with the different barbell, dumbbell, and pulley exercises, including EZ curl bars, to find out which exercises you can do without provoking your forearm problem.

Overwork

Question: I love bodybuilding, have been doing it for years, but every time I complete a really heavy workout, I get either a sore throat or a cold, or a case of the runs (diarrhea). I desperately want to be a champ. Help me, please.

Answer: You are overworking. You need to backtrack a little. Make your workouts less exhausting. Then gradually build up the intensity again. Do it slowly. Do not miss several workouts and then suddenly go all out. This would bring back your problems. Overwork puts the system in shock and is counterproductive to successful bodybuilding.

Sets

Question: I would like to know why some bodybuilders—Arnold Schwarzenegger, Casey Viator, Frank Zane, to name just a few—perform 20 or more sets per body part and still exercise with a great deal of intensity, while others advocate the same high intensity but only 1 or 2 sets. How come?

Answer: Other things being equal, 20 sets are more demanding than 1 or 2 sets. In fact, 20 sets are more demanding than 19 sets. There are, however, also a lot of other variables, such as the amount of time that is available for training, the ability of one's body to recuperate, the tolerance of one's metabolism and nervous system for strenuous and prolonged exercise—the list goes on. One thing is certain: doing more sets is entirely useless if it involves overtraining and not fully recuperating between workouts. This is why the Mentzer System is so popular: It is based on the fact that you only need a minimal number of sets (1–2) to zap the muscles into growth.

What is needed for regular gains is progression. Intensity is of prime importance, but not everyone can keep on increasing intensity, workout after workout. The next and probably easiest step is to increase the number of sets. The problem here is that the more sets you do, the more the muscle cells are stimulated, but it is very much a matter of diminishing returns. In other words, 20 sets per body part are better than 10 sets, but only *fractionally*. You have to perform a great many more sets to effect smaller and smaller benefits—provided you recuperate between workouts. Without full recovery, you'll drive yourself, not to the top of bodybuilding, but into the ground.

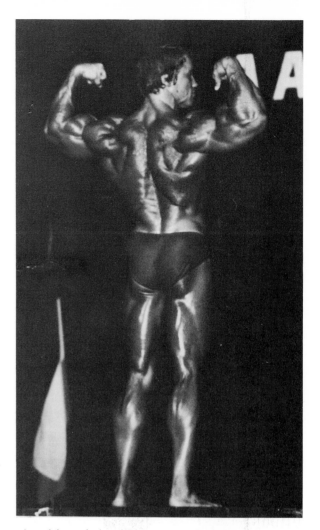

Arnold maximized his enormous potential.

A Joule?

Question: I am naturally heavy, so am constantly on a diet and buy just about every book on the subject. Recently I came upon a new word, which I just don't understand. Could you please tell me what a *joule* is?

Answer: Joules (J) are going to be used to measure energy. One calorie is equal to 4.2 joules, and 100 joules is a kilojoule. One million joules will be known as a megajoule. For the time being, you may as well stick to calories—everyone else probably will.

Stretch Marks

Question: I'm only a young bodybuilder (26 years old), but I am worried because

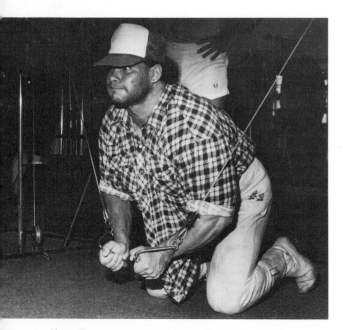

Kneeling crossover pulleys, Barbarian-style.

I am getting stretch marks at the side of my chest, and even on my arms. It is so bad that I may even quit training. What do you suggest I do to get rid of them?

Answer: Some people think stretch marks are caused by growing too fast: your muscles are growing faster than your skin. In fact, faulty nutrition should take much of the blame. If you do not feed your body the essential nutrients it needs, then it will rob nutrients from the least essential organs, often the skin. This makes the skin less elastic and more likely to tear under strain. To help avoid stretch marks, you should supplement your body with a good B-Complex supplement, vitamins A, D, and E, and pantothenic acid. With stretch marks that have already occurred, you can try and minimize the damage by rubbing them with Vitamin E oil (the d-alpha tocopherol type). This helps to dissolve the keloids in the scar tissue and will minimize the unsightly effect. You can have stretch marks removed surgically, but the results are not always satisfactory.

Belts

Question: Do I need a lifting belt? I see that many bodybuilders wear these in their training, but I do not want to waste my money if a belt is not really necessary.

Answer: Most bodybuilding, like weightlifting, involves overload training. Heavy training can put a stress on the lower back. It is definitely advisable to use a belt in all overhead lifts, rowing, deadlifts, and all forms of squats. A belt diffuses the strain of heavy poundage and so reduces the chance of injury to the lower back. A belt is like an additional set of waistline muscles. Look at the seasoned squatter who never uses a belt: his tummy is way out to here!

A belt will not only keep you tight for your exercises and help to ward off injury, it will also greatly add to your strength once you get accustomed to it. Movements like the barbell or dumbbell press, deadlifts, and squats will improve 10 percent or more. Remember that a belt doesn't have to be drawn tight all the time. Most trainers wear it loose and only tighten it up (very tight) just before an important set of heavy exercises. Immediately after completing that set they loosen it again. Belts are *not* needed for bench press or abdominal exercises.

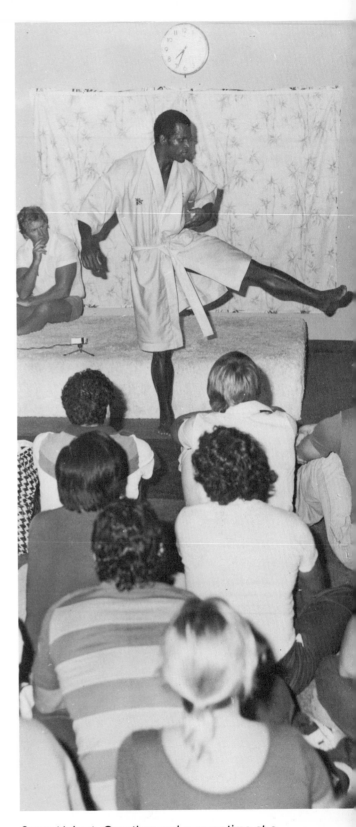

Serge Nubret: Question and answer time at a seminar in Australia.

30
THE GUYS
AT THE TOP
Who Won
Which Title
When

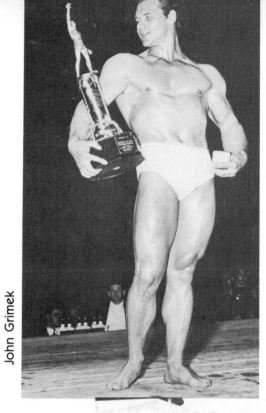

John Grimek

Dennis Tinerino

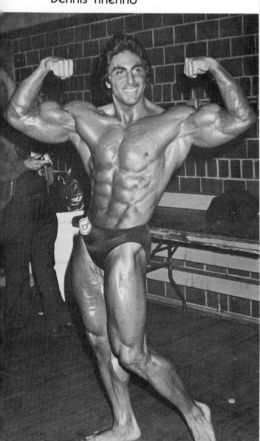

Reg Park

Sergio Oliva

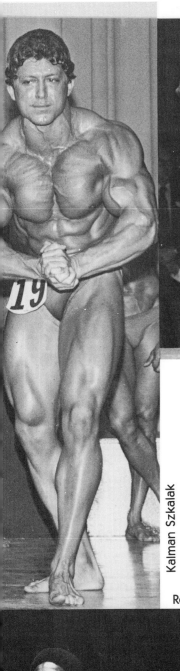

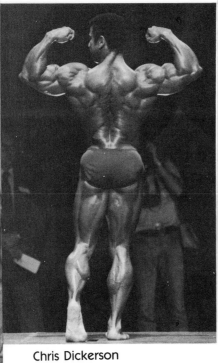

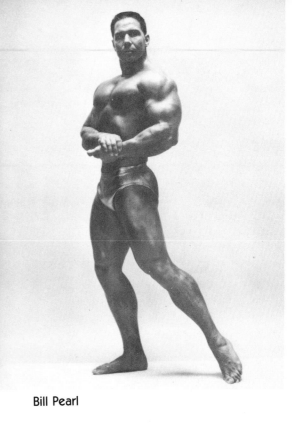

Chris Dickerson

Bill Pearl

Arnold Schwarzenegger

Kalman Szkalak

Robbie Robinson and Frank Zane

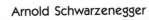

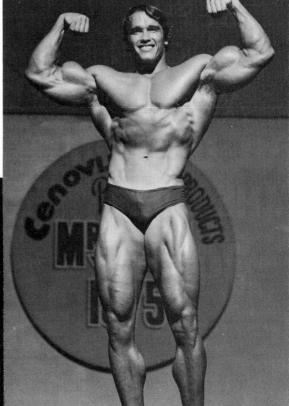

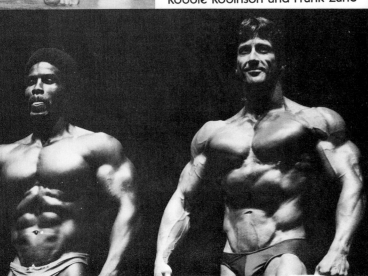

AAU TITLE WINNERS

Mr. America

1938　Bert Goodrich
1939　Roland Essmaker
1940　John Grimek
　　　Frank Leight

1941　John Grimek
　　　Chuck Deutsch

1942　Frank Leight
1943　Jules Bacon
1944　Steve Stanko
1945　Clarence Ross
　　　Harold Zinkin
　　　K.D. Graham
　　　E. Rodriquez
　　　Phil Courtois

1946　Alan Stephan
1947　Steve Reeves
　　　Eric Pedersen
　　　Joe Lauriano

1948　George Eiferman
　　　Jack Delinger

1949　Jack Delinger
1950　John Farbotnik
　　　Melvin Wells
　　　Roy Hilligen

1951　Roy Hilligen
　　　Malcolm Brenner
　　　Marvin Eder
　　　George Paine ⎫ tied
　　　Pepper Gomez ⎭

1952　Jim Park
　　　Malcolm Brenner
　　　George Paine
　　　Don Van Fleteran

1953　Bill Pearl
　　　Dick DuBois
　　　Irvin Koszewski
　　　Steve Klisanin
　　　George Paine

1954　Dick Du Bois
　　　Gene Bohaty
　　　Irvin Koszewski
　　　George Paine
　　　Lud Shusterich

1955　Steve Klisanin
　　　Ray Schaeffer
　　　Vic Seipke ⎫
　　　Don Van Fleteran ⎬ tied
　　　Harry Johnson ⎭

1956　Ray Schaeffer
1957　Ron Lacy
1958　Tom Sansone
1959　Harry Johnson
　　　Ray Routledge
　　　Pete Ganios
　　　George Orlando
　　　Vern Weaver

1960　Lloyd Lerille
　　　Ray Routledge
　　　Joe Lazzaro
　　　Bill Stathes
　　　Joe Abbenda

1961　Ray Routledge
　　　Joe Abbenda
　　　Franklin Jones
　　　Harold Poole
　　　Bill Golumdick

1962　Joe Abbenda
　　　Harold Poole
　　　Hugo Labra
　　　Vern Weaver
　　　Vic Seipke

1963　Vern Weaver
　　　Harold Poole
　　　Craig Whitehead
　　　John Gourgott
　　　William Seno

1964　Val Vasilieff
　　　John Gourgott
　　　Randy Watson
　　　William Seno
　　　Craig Whitehead

1965　Jerry Daniels
　　　Bob Gajda
　　　Randy Watson
　　　Sergio Oliva
　　　Charles Estes

1966　Bob Gajda
　　　Sergio Oliva
　　　Ralph Kroger
　　　Randy Watson
　　　Jim Haislop

1967　Dennis Tinerino
　　　Jim Haislop
　　　Wil Whitaker
　　　Ralph Kroger
　　　Boyer Coe

1968　Jim Haislop
　　　Boyer Coe
　　　Chris Dickerson
　　　Ken Waller
　　　Chuck Collras

1969　Boyer Coe
　　　Chris Dickerson
　　　Ken Waller

1970　Chris Dickerson
　　　Ken Waller
　　　Casey Viator

1971　Casey Viator
　　　Pete Grymkowski
　　　Bill St. John
　　　Ed Corney
　　　Carl Smith

1972　Steve Michalik
　　　Pete Grymkowski
　　　Jim Morris
　　　Bill St. John
　　　Ken Covington

1973　Jim Morris
　　　Pete Grymkowski
　　　Anibal Lopez
　　　Paul Hill
　　　Willie Johnson

1974	Ron Thompson		
	Paul Hill		
	Doug Beaver		
	Willie Johnson		
	Ralph Kroger		

1974   Ron Thompson
      Paul Hill
      Doug Beaver
      Willie Johnson
      Ralph Kroger

1975   Dale Adrian
      Clinton Beyerle
      Pat Neve
      Mike Dayton
      Robbie Robinson

1976   Kalman Szkalak
      Dave Johns
      Clinton Beyerle
      Joe Means
      Pat Neve

1977   Dave Johns
      Manuel Perry
      Ron Tuefel
      Clinton Beyerle
      Dr. C.F. Smith

1978   Tony Pearson
      Ron Tuefel
      Manuel Perry

1979   Ray Mentzer
      Gary Leonard
      Ron Tuefel

1980   Gary Leonard
      Bronston Austin, Jr.
      Richard Baldwin
      Ken Passariello

1981   Tim Belknap
      Lance Dreher
      James Youngblood
      Ken Passariello

1982   Rufus Howard
      Phil Rhode
      Jesse Gautreaux
      Mike Sable

Junior Mr. America

1944   Steve Stanko
1945   Joseph Lauriano
1946   Everett Sinderoff
1947   Edward J. Simons
1948   Harry Smith
1949   Val Pasqua
1950   John Farbotnik
1951   George Paine
1952   Malcolm Brenner
1953   Steve Klisanin
1954   Gene Bohaty } tied
      Harry Johnson
1955   Vic Seipke
1956   Ray Schaeffer
1957   Jim Dugger
1958   Tom Sansone (East)
      Ray Routledge (West)
1959   Elmo Santiago
1960   Joe Lazzaro (East)
      Frank A. Quinn (South)
      Gail Crick (Southwest)
      Hugo Labra (West)
1961   Joe Simon (East)
      Ronnie Russell (Southeast)
      John Gourgott (South)
      Lou Wolter (Midwest)
      Harold Poole (Central)
      Franklin Jones (West)
1962   Joseph Abbenda (East)
      Billy Lemacks (South)
      Tuny Monday (Midwest)
1963   Randy Watson
1964   John Decola
1965   Jerry Daniels
1966   Sergio Oliva
1967   Dennis Tinerino
1968   Jim Haislop
1969   Boyer Coe
1970   Chris Dickerson
1971   Casey Viator
1972   Pete Grymkowski
1973   Paul Hill
1974   Ron Thompson
1975   Willie Johnson
1976   Dave Johns
1977   Mario Nieves
1978   Tony Pearson
1979   Robert Jodkiewicz
1980   Ernie Santiago
1981   Marty Vranicar
1982   Michael Antonio

Teenage Mr. America

1958   John Gourgott
1959   Joe Abbenda
1960   Jerry Doettrell (East)
      Gil Dimeglio (Central)
      John Corvello (West)
1961   Steve Boyer (East)
      John Piscareta (Midwest)
1962   Michael Liscio (East)
      Mickey Majors (Midwest)
1963   Jerry Daniels
1964   Bud Schosek
1965   Dennis Tinerino
1966   Boyer Coe
1967   Mike Dayton
1968   Ken Covington
1969   Bob Gallucci
1970   Casey Viator
1971   Scott Pace
1972   Sammie Willis
1973   Joe Ugolik
1974   Dan Tobol
1975   Ron Tuefel
1976   Mike Torschia
1977   Jim Yasenchock
1978   Rudy Hermosillo
1979   Lee Haney
1980   Danny Berumen
1981   Michael Quinn

Over-40 Mr. America

1976   Vic Seipke
1977   Kent Kuehn
1978   Earl Maynard
1979   Phil Outlaw
1980   Paul Love
1981   O.J. Smith

Mr. USA

1964	Mike Ferraro
1965	Bob Gajda
1966	Dennis Tinerino
1967	Jim Haislop
1968	Chris Dickerson
1969	Ken Waller
1970	Casey Viator
1971	Steve Michalik
1972	Jim Morris
1973	Paul Hill
1974	Pat Neve
1975	Clinton Beyerle
1976	Manuel Perry
1977	Rod Koontz
1978	Ron Tuefel
1979	Robert Reis
1980	Dave Rogers
1981	Jesse Gautreaux

Junior Mr. USA

1965	Dennis Tinerino
1966	Chris Dickerson
1967	James Morris
1968	Boyer Coe
1969	Ken Waller
1970	Carl Smith
1971	Pete Grymkowski
1972	Ron Thompson
1973	Paul Hill
1974	Dave Johns
1975	Floyd Odom
1976	Joe Means
1977	Dave Rogers
1978	Tony Pearson
1979	Jim Seitzer
1980	Ernie Santiago
1981	Robert Coburn

Teenage Mr. USA

1975	Steve Shields
1976	Steve Borodinsky
1977	Rudy Hermosillo
1978	Casey Kucharyk
1979	Joe Fulco
1980	John Taylor
1981	Konstantine Spanoudis

Over-40 Mr. USA

1979	Paul Yazolino
1980	Don Len
1981	Art Peacock

Mr. California

1946	Steve Reeves
1951	Roy Hilligen
1953	Bill Pearl
1955	Jerry Ross
1960	Larry Scott
1961	Hugo Labra
1963	Don Howorth
1964	Joe Nista
1965	John Corvello
1966	Ralph Kroger
1969	Paul Love
1970	Chris Dickerson
1972	Ed Corney
1973	Mike Besikoff
1974	Scott Wilson
1975	Dale Adrian
1976	Kalman Szkalak
1977	Dave Johns
1978	Ron Tuefel
1979	Larry Jackson
1980	Rory Leidelmeyer
1981	Ed Zajac
1982	Doug Brignole

Mr. World

1970	Ken Waller (amateur)
	Arnold Schwarzenegger (pro)
1971	Albert Beckles
1972	Paul Grant
1973	Ron Thompson
1974	Roy Duval
1975	Ian Lawrence
1976	Bertil Fox

FHI Title Winners

Mr. Universe

1947	Steve Stanko
1950	John Farbotnik
1954	Tommy Kono
1955	Tommy Kono
1957	Tommy Kono
1959	Guy Mierczuk
1961	Tommy Kono
1963	Ahmed El-Guindi
1964	Ahmed El-Guindi
1965	Bill March
1966	Bob Gajda

NBBA Title Winners

Natural Mr. America

1978	Tyronne Youngs (amateur)
	Dennis Tinerino (pro)
1979	Ron Magnum (amateur)
	Tyronne Youngs (pro)
	Doug Brignole (teenage)
	Jerry Englebert (over-40)
1980	Chuck Buser (amateur)
	Rod Koontz (pro)
1981	Eddie Love

Mr. America

1981	Bob Gallucci
	Bohdan Narolsky (teenage)
	Jim Karas (over-40)
1982	Mike Ashley
	Lance Scurvin (teenage)
	Reg Lewis (over-40)

NABBA Title Winners

Mr. Universe

1948	John Grimek
1950	Steve Reeves
1951	Reg Park

Amateur

1952	Mohammed Nasr
1953	Bill Pearl
1954	Enrico Thomas
1955	Mickey Hargitay
1956	Ray Schaeffer
1957	John Lees
1958	Earl Clark
1959	Len Sell
1960	Henry Downs
1961	Ray Routledge
1962	Joe Abbenda
1963	Tom Sansone
1964	John Hewlett
1965	Elmo Santiago
1966	Chester Yorton
1967	Arnold Schwarzenegger
1968	Dennis Tinerino
1969	Boyer Coe
1970	Frank Zane
1971	Ken Waller
1972	Elias Petsas
1973	Chris Dickerson
1974	Roy Duval
1975	Ian Lawrence
1976	Shigeru Sugita
1977	Bertil Fox
1978	Dave Johns
1979	Ahmet Enunlu
1980	Bill Richardson
1981	John Brown
1982	John Brown

Professional

1952	Juan Ferrero
1953	Arnold Tyson
1954	Jim Park
1955	Leo Robert
1956	Jack Delinger
1957	Arthur Robin
1958	Reg Park
1959	Bruce Randall
1960	Paul Wynter
1961	Bill Pearl
1962	Len Sell
1963	Joe Abbenda
1964	Earl Maynard
1965	Reg Park
1966	Paul Wynter
1967	Bill Pearl
1968	Arnold Schwarzenegger
1969	Arnold Schwarzenegger
1970	Arnold Schwarzenegger
1971	Bill Pearl
1972	Frank Zane
1973	Boyer Coe
1974	Chris Dickerson
1975	Boyer Coe
1976	Serge Nubret
1977	Tony Emmott
1978	Bertil Fox
1979	Bertil Fox
1980	Tony Pearson
1981	Robbie Robinson
1982	Eduardo Kowak

Mr. Britain

1930	W.T. Coggins
1931	C. Coster
1932	W.T. Coggins
1933	S. Ingleson
1934	W. Bower
1935	W. Purchon
1936	W. Archer
1937	O. Heidenstam
1938	T. Moreland
1939	H. Loveday
1940	G. Allan
1941	K. Paton
1942	*No Contest*
1943	Don Dorans
1944	Gordon MacKay
1945	Bill Beaumont
1946	Charles Curzon
1947	Jim Elliot
1948	Charles Jarrett
1949	Reg Park
1950	Hubert Thomas
1951	Dennis Stallard
1952	Mervynne Cotter
1953	John Lees
1954	Wally Wright
1955	Bill Parkinson
1956	Henry Downs
1957	Len Sell
1958	John Hewlett
1959	Tony Rothwell
1960	Adrian Heryet
1961	Dave Stroud
1962	Ted Guttridge
1963	Paul Nash
1964	Terry Parkinson
1965	John Citrone
1966	John Citrone
1967	Wilf Sylvester
1968	Brian Eastman
1969	Frank Richard
1970	Albert Beckles
1971	Albert Beckles
1972	Paul Grant
1973	Roy Duval
1974	Eddie McDonough
1975	Ian Lawrence
1976	Bertil Fox
1977	Eddie McDonough
1978	Bill Richardson
1979	Terry Phillips
1980	Graham Brogden
1981	Eddie Millar
1982	Ian Dowe

IFBB Contest Winners

Mr. America
1949	Alan Stephan
1959	Chuck Sipes
1960	Gene Shuey
1962	Larry Scott
1963	Reg Lewis
1964	Harold Poole
1965	Dave Draper
1966	Chet Yorton
1967	Don Howorth
1968	Frank Zane
1969	John Decola
1970	Mike Katz
1971	Ken Waller
1972	Ed Corney
1973	Lou Ferrigno
1974	Bob Birdsong
1975	Robbie Robinson
1976	Mike Mentzer

Mr. World
1962	Jose Castaneda Lence
1963	Jorge Brisco
1965	Kingsley Poitier
1966	Sergio Oliva
1967	Rick Wayne
1968	Chuck Sipes
1969	Frank Zane
1970	Dave Draper
1971	Franco Columbu
1972	Mike Katz
1973	Ken Waller
1974	Bill Grant
1975	Robbie Robinson
1977	Darcey Beccles

1982 NPC Title Winners

Mr. America
Lee Haney
Moses Maldonado
Dale Ruplinger
James Gaubert
Junior: Lee Haney
Teenage: Doyle Washington
Over-40: Bob McGinty

Mr. USA
Dale Ruplinger
Junior: Phil Outlaw
Over-40: Dave Berman

Mr. California
John Jordon

Mr. Universe
1959	Eddie Silvestre
1961	Chuck Sipes
1962	George Eiferman
1963	Harold Poole
1964	Larry Scott
1965	Earl Maynard
1966	Dave Draper
1967	Sergio Oliva
1968	Frank Zane
1969	Arnold Schwarzenegger
1970	Arnold Schwarzenegger
1971	Albert Beckles
1972	Ed Corney
1973	Lou Ferrigno
1974	Lou Ferrigno
1975	Ken Waller
1976	Mohamed Makkawy (*light*)
	Robbie Robinson (*middle*)
	Roger Walker (*heavy*)
1977	Danny Padilla (*light*)
	Roy Callendar (*middle*)
	Kalman Szkalak (*heavy*)
1978	Carlos Rodriquez (*light*)
	Tom Platz (*middle*)
	Mike Mentzer (*heavy*)
1979	Renato Bertagna (*light*)
	Roy Duval (*middle*)
	Samir Bannout (*light-heavy*)
	Jusup Wilkosz (*heavy*)

1980	Heinz Sallmayer (*light*)
	Jorma Raty (*middle*)
	Johnny Fuller (*light-heavy*)
	Hubert Metz (*heavy*)
1981	Ken Passariello (*light*)
	Gerard Buinoud (*middle*)
	Jacques Neuville (*light-heavy*)
	Lance Dreher (*heavy*)
1982	James Gaubert (*light*)
	Dale Ruplinger (*middle*)
	Ahmet Enunlu (*light-heavy*)
	Lee Haney (*heavy*)

Mr. Europe
1981	Jose Rabanal (France) (*light*)
	Anton Holic (Czech.) (*middle*)
	Libor Minarik (Czech.) (*light-heavy*)
	Gunnar Rosbo (Norway) (*heavy*)
1982	Herman Hoffend (Germany) (*light*)
	Erwin Note (Belgium) (*middle*)
	Libor Minarik (Czech.) (*light-heavy*)
	Berry Derney (*heavy*)

Mr. International
1974	Lou Ferrigno
1976	Robbie Robinson
1977	Mohamed Makkawy
1978	Joe Nazzario
1979	Greg DeFerro
1980	Andreas Cahling
1981	Scott Wilson

Pro Mr. Universe
1975	Bob Birdsong
1978	Roy Callendar
1979	Roy Callendar
1980	Jusup Wilkosz
1981	Dennis Tinerino

Mr. Olympia

1965	Larry Scott
1966	Larry Scott
1967	Sergio Oliva
1968	Sergio Oliva
1969	Sergio Oliva
1970	Arnold Schwarzenegger
1971	Arnold Schwarzenegger
1972	Arnold Schwarzenegger
1973	Arnold Schwarzenegger
1974	Arnold Schwarzenegger

Under 200
Franco Columbu
Frank Zane
Over 200
Arnold Schwarzenegger
Lou Ferrigno

1975	Arnold Schwarzenegger

Under 200
Franco Columbu
Ed Corney
Albert Beckles
Over 200
Arnold Schwarzenegger
Serge Nubret
Lou Ferrigno

1976	Franco Columbu

Under 200
Franco Columbu
Frank Zane
Boyer Coe
Over 200
Ken Waller
Mike Katz

1977	Frank Zane
	Robbie Robinson
	Ed Corney
	Boyer Coe
	Ken Waller

1978	Frank Zane
	Robbie Robinson
	Roy Callendar
	Boyer Coe
	Kalman Szkalak
	Danny Padilla

1979	Frank Zane
	Mike Mentzer
	Boyer Coe
	Robbie Robinson
	Dennis Tinerino
	Chris Dickerson

1980	Arnold Schwarzenegger
	Chris Dickerson
	Frank Zane
	Boyer Coe
	Mike Mentzer
	Roger Walker

1981	Franco Columbu
	Chris Dickerson
	Tom Platz
	Roy Callendar
	Danny Padilla
	Jusup Wilkosz

1982	Chris Dickerson
	Frank Zane
	Casey Viator
	Samir Bannout
	Albert Beckles
	Tom Platz

WABBA
Contest Winners

Mr. World

1977	Ahmet Enunlu *(amateur)*
	Sergio Oliva *(pro)*
1978	Ahmet Enunlu
1979	Tony Pearson
1980	Eduardo Kowak *(amateur)*
	Sergio Oliva *(pro)*
1982	Eduardo Kowak

Pro World Cup

1981	Sergio Oliva

Mr. Europe

1978	Bill Richardson
1979	Terry Phillips
1980	Bill Richardson

Long Beach

Sergio Oliva *(pro)*
Bill Richardson *(amateur)*

Mr. America

Vince Fillipelli
Mike Steffick *(teenage)*
Lou Kushner *(over-40)*

WBBG
Title Winners

1967	Harold Poole
1968	Harold Poole
1969	Johnny Maldonado
1970	Rick Wayne
1971	Peter Caputo
1972	Bill Grant
1973	Chris Dickerson
1974	Warren Frederick
1975	Ralph Kroger
1976	Scott Wilson
1977	Don Ross
1978	Anibal Lopez
1979	Tommy Aybar

Mr. World

1971	Boyer Coe
1972	Boyer Coe
1973	Boyer Coe
1974	Boyer Coe
1975	Boyer Coe
1976	Tony Emmott
1977	Serge Nubret
1978	Anibal Lopez
1979	Tony Pearson

Mr. Olympus

1975	Sergio Oliva
1976	Sergio Oliva
1977	Serge Nubret
1978	Sergio Oliva
1979	Tony Pearson

Professional Contest Winners

1978 Gold's Classic-World Cup
Robbie Robinson

Night of Champions (NYC)
Robbie Robinson

1979 Night of Champions
Robbie Robinson

Southern Cup
Mike Mentzer

Pittsburgh Pro Cup
Robbie Robinson

Diamond Cup (Vancouver)
Roy Callendar

Best in the World Show
Robbie Robinson

Canada Cup
Chris Dickerson

1980 Professional Grand Prix
Florida: Chris Dickerson
Louisiana: Casey Viator
California: Chris Dickerson
Pittsburgh: Casey Viator
New York: Chris Dickerson
Overall: Chris Dickerson (74 pts)
　　　　Casey Viator (63 pts)
　　　　Robbie Robinson (44 pts)
　　　　Boyer Coe (33 pts)
　　　　Samir Bannout (24 pts)

Canada Cup
Chris Dickerson

1981 Professional Grand Prix
California: Chris Dickerson
Louisiana: Chris Dickerson
Washington, D.C.: Chris Dickerson
New England: Albert Beckles
New York: Chris Dickerson
Overall: Chris Dickerson

World Grand Prix (Montreal)
Boyer Coe

Note: Two other Grand Prix contests were held in Europe (Belgium and Wales) and Boyer Coe won both. If these contests are counted in the overall standings, then Boyer Coe was the overall Grand Prix winner.

World Cup (Atlantic City)
Boyer Coe (307 pts, the highest score ever attained in an IFBB contest)

1982 Night of Champions (NYC)
Albert Beckles

IFBB Pro World Championship
Albert Beckles
Boyer Coe
Johnny Fuller
Mohamed Makkawy
Roy Callendar

1983 Night of Champions (NYC)
Lee Haney
Greg DeFerro
Albert Beckles
John Fuller
John Terelli

INDEX